HEALTH CARE IN AMERICA

Essays in Social History

EDITED BY

SUSAN REVERBY *and*
DAVID ROSNER

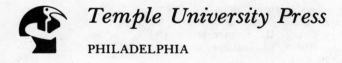

Temple University Press

PHILADELPHIA

Temple University Press, Philadelphia 19122
© 1979 by Temple University. All rights reserved
Published 1979
Printed in the United States of America

Library of Congress Cataloging in Publication Data

Main entry under title:

Health care in America.

    Includes bibliographical references and index.
    1. Social medicine—United States—History—
Addresses, essays, lectures. 2. Medical care—
United States—History—Addresses, essays, lectures.
I. Reverby, Susan. II. Rosner, David, 1947-
[DNLM: 1. History of medicine, Modern—United
States. WZ70 AA1 H4]
RA418.3.U6H42   362.1'0973   79-14613
ISBN 0-87722-153-7 cloth
ISBN 0-87722-171-5 paper

Contents

Contributors

E. RICHARD BROWN teaches in the Behavioral Sciences and Health Education division of the U.C.L.A. School of Public Health. His book, *Rockfeller Medicine Men: Medicine and Capitalism in America,* has just been published by the University of California Press.

ROBERT CRAWFORD is in the Department of Political Science at the University of Illinois, Chicago Circle. He is currently engaged in research on the role of industry in cost control politics and industrial health policies for workers.

VIRGINIA G. DRACHMAN is in the History Department at Tufts University. She is presently at the Radcliffe Institute in Cambridge, working on a study of the women's medical movement.

LEON FINK is a member of the History Department at the University of North Carolina at Chapel Hill. He and Brian Greenberg are currently completing a larger study of hospital unionization efforts.

BRIAN GREENBERG is in the Department of History at Princeton University. He is the author of other works in labor history and is working on a larger study of Local 1199 with Leon Fink.

JUDITH WALZER LEAVITT teaches in the History of Medicine Department and Women's Studies at the University of Wisconsin in Madison. She has co-edited *Medicine Without Doctors: Home Health Care in American History* (1977) and *Sickness and Health in America: Readings in the History of Medicine and Public Health* (1978), and is completing an historical study of public health in urban America.

Contributors

GERALD E. MARKOWITZ is in the Department of History at John J. College of Criminal Justice at the City University of New York. His present research is on the W. P. A. during the Depression.

LAWRENCE G. MILLER has written on various aspects of medical history. He is in the Department of Medicine at the Massachusetts General Hospital.

SUSAN REVERBY is in the American and New England Studies Progam at Boston University. She is the co-editor of *America's Working Women, A Documentary History* (1976) and presently is studying the rationalization of hospital nursing in the United States.

BARBARA G. ROSENKRANTZ is in the Department of the History of Science and in the School of Public Health at Harvard University. She is the author of *Public Health and the State, Changing Views in Massachusetts, 1842-1936* (1972) and numerous other books and articles in the field of the history of public health and medicine.

DAVID ROSNER teaches in the Baruch College-Mt. Sinai School of Medicine Program in Health Administration and in the Baruch College Department of History. He is completing a study of the development of an urban health care system during the Progressive Era.

MARTHA H. VERBRUGGE is in the Department of History at Bucknell University. Her research concerns female health and education in nineteenth-century Boston.

MARIS A. VINOVSKIS is a member of the Department of History and the Center for Political Studies of the Institute for Social Research at the University of Michigan. He and Barbara Rosenkrantz are working on a larger project on antebellum mental asylums.

MORRIS J. VOGEL is in the Department of History at Temple University. His book, tentatively titled *The American General Hospital: A Social History,* will be published by the University of Chicago Press.

PART I

INTRODUCTION

SUSAN REVERBY
and DAVID ROSNER

1 *Beyond "the Great Doctors"*

This volume is a contribution toward a social history of health care in America. We purposefully use the term "health care" rather than "medicine" because these essays examine the social relations of health care, rather than the activity and intellectual concerns of physicians alone. "The history of medicine is infinitely more than the history of the great doctors and their books," wrote Henry E. Sigerist, a prominent medical historian, nearly a half century ago.[1] In light of our recognition of the complexity of health care delivery and the post-World War II growth of the health industry, this dictum is now even more relevant.

A history that both illuminates health policy concerns and explores the subtleties of medicine's past is being built with the questions and tools of what is called the "new social history." This history explicitly examines the growth and transformation of society's structures, institutions, and culture. Its current formulation has been shaped in part by contemporary political struggles.[2] The Civil Rights, Anti-War, and Women's movements all focused the historian's attentions on class and familial relations and the different historical experiences of minorities, women, and the working class. In the absence of an abundance of the usual written sources to explore this history, social historians have turned to social science methodology, computer technology, and new sources of data such as manuscript censuses, city directories, and tax lists.

The social history perspective raises important questions when applied to medical and health care issues. Some of these questions concern the social and political responses to disease, the social epidemiology of health and illness, the changing definition and importance of professionalism, the ideological and social control aspects of medicine, and the social role of health care institutions.[3]

Until recently these social concerns were not central to the history of medicine because the field focused primarily on the unfolding of medical science and "the ideas that have animated physicians."[4] This dominant medical history tradition reflects both a pervasive societal faith in the potential and efficacy of medical science and the fact that much of this history was written by physicians. As Owsei Temkin has noted, "the history of medicine . . . [was] conceived as a march of progress culminating in the present state of superior medical and scientific knowledge."[5] With the growing understanding of both the social causation of health and disease and the way in which science is embedded in a society's social relations, however, historians have begun to reanalyze medical history.

The essays in this volume, while diverse in their analytical frameworks, address three themes of central concern to the health field:

(1) the shifting boundaries between professional and lay control over the definition of health and disease;

(2) the social and economic consequences of the changing locus of health care delivery; and

(3) the complex relationship between workers, professionals, and health care institutions.

The linking of contemporary medical issues with the writing of history has a long tradition. At certain historical moments, medical history was valued as a way to keep physicians in touch with humanistic concerns in the face of an increasingly technological and specialized medical practice. At other times, medical history has been marshalled in support of different positions in the battles over medical and health care reforms. In the following pages we will briefly trace the close relationship between the history of medicine and medicine, emphasizing the political nature of this alliance.[6] We do this to ground the new social history of health care in its past.

Until the end of the nineteenth century many of the theoretical and practical formulations of medical practitioners were derived from history.[7] An understanding of the Ancients, their therapeutic regimens and theoretical justifications, lent credence to various medical practices. Hippocrates, Aristotle, and Galen dot the pages of pre-twentieth-century medical writings just as references to current research appear in this year's publications.[8] Medical history was written by practitioners for practitioners.

With the development of science as the dominant ideology and material base of medicine, history lost its function as medicine's source of authority. In medicine, as in other aspects of American life, innovation, progress, and scientific advance, rather than recourse to ancient authorities, became highly valued. In centers where this scientific medicine was most advanced, the history of medicine took on a new function.

Nowhere was this clearer than at the medical and nursing schools organized at Johns Hopkins University in Baltimore in the 1880s. The men and women of the new scientific generation at Hopkins were aware that medicine and nursing entailed more than scientific knowledge and technical skills. With the growing importance of science, they were deeply concerned that the art of medical and nursing practice might be lost. For them, the art entailed clinical decision-making, "bedside manner," the development of the physician's and nurse's "character," and a sensitivity to the patient's humanity. They saw the training of their students in this "humanism" as an essential counterweight to the possible dehumanizing effects of the new science. For them, the study of history was the linchpin that could hold together both the science and the art of medicine and nursing.[9] Harvey Cushing, the famed surgeon, later eloquently voiced this motive for his generation's abiding concern with history:

> In the modern development of the physician into a scientist have we not lost something precious that may without risk of pedantry be brought back to Medicine? Not only has the art of healing, *die Heilkunst,* come more and more to be lost sight of as the doctor arrives at his diagnosis in the laboratory rather than at the bedside, but less and less does he care to be reminded that poetry, history, rhetoric and the humanities once had close kinship with natural philosophy when *Doctores Medicinae* took the leadership among the *Artisti.*[10]

The history of medicine functioned as an excursion into moral philosophy and ethics and as a unifying theme for an increasingly specialized profession. This history was to be, as George Sarton would later argue for the history of science, a new humanism that did not reject but rather embraced science and practical knowledge.[11]

Thus, as soon as the nursing and medical schools opened at Hopkins, history lectures were given. In addition, William Osler, who headed the Hopkins medical department, merged medical history with his daily medical teaching on rounds. As he described it:

> A case of exopthalmic goitre comes in—the question at once is put, Who was Graves? Who was Parry? Who was Basedow? Of course the student does not know; he is told to bring, on another day, the original article, and he is given five or ten minutes in which to read a brief historical note.[12]

"In this way," Harvey Cushing wrote, "many students who unquestionably would have sidestepped a formal course of lectures became unconsciously impregnated" with history.[13] For those more consciously interested in history, a Johns Hopkins Hospital Historical Club was organized at which formal papers, later published in the hospital's *Bulletin,* were presented.

This generation's approach to history places medical ideas in a cultural context, although to the modern reader its erudite style appears inaccessible and flowery. In addition, the students acquired a peculiar vision of medical history—rooted deep in historical time but focused narrowly on specific individuals and discoveries.[14] The Oslerian method of teaching the history of medicine was also predicated upon medical schools' having a faculty steeped in history.[15]

Ironically, as this history strove to bind the student to his past, it severed these tenuous ties. As an intellectual history, dependent upon a knowledge of Greek and Latin and the skills imparted by a classical education, its lessons for the practically oriented medical student became less and less clear. Even when this history examined medicine in its American context, it appeared to have little to teach the new science-trained medical student, who was more concerned with breaks than continuities with the past. Similarly, it was assumed that only a physician, with the technical knowledge of medicine and an understanding of the subtleties of medical culture, could be a medical historian.

Medical students were therefore isolated from general currents in history.

Medical history was becoming extraneous to medical education despite its proponents' attempts to make apparent its usefullness. Survey after survey in the 1900s through the 1920s drew dismal pictures of haphazard courses and occasional lectures in most medical schools.[16] Yet a small coterie of physicians and medical educators banded together to give medical history an institutional form. In the 1920s medical history journals appeared sporadically and the American Association for the History of Medicine was organized.[17] In 1926 the interest in medical history on the part of the Johns Hopkins faculty culminated in the appointment of the then retiring William Henry Welch to a chair in the history of medicine and the beginning of plans for an institute in the history of medicine. Thus, the lack of widespread interest in the history of medicine pushed its proponents to establish an institutional base.

The relationship between history and medicine took on a new meaning with the appointment of Henry E. Sigerist as Welch's replacement as the head of the Johns Hopkins Institute of the History of Medicine in 1932. A physician-philologist, trained as a medical historian under Karl Sudhoff at the University of Leipzig's Institute of the History of Medicine, Sigerist professionalized the history of medicine in America. He combined the academic classical tradition with a new definition of the art of medicine. While previously the art had been seen as medical humanism, centered on the doctor-patient relationship, Sigerist expanded its boundaries to include social and political phenomena. He shared with the earlier medical generation a belief that:

> Modern medicine had become so specialized and so technical that some place had to be established in medical schools where medicine would be studied, not from the specialist's point of view, but as a whole, as an entity—and in its relationship to the other sciences, and to society as a whole.[18]

His history of medicine had an additional element that Sigerist defined as "sociological," the study of the development of socioeconomic structures of various civilizations and their relationship to health care.[19] Sigerist sought, in his voluminous historical writings, to place medicine in "a matrix that was at once cultural, social and economic."[20]

Although his historical work was not always overtly political, he saw much of it as part of a larger political and educational effort to transform the health care system.[21] His history was to serve two functions: "It should give us a more complete picture of the development of civilization and . . . should make us aware [of] where we come from in medicine, at what point we are standing today, and in what direction we are marching."[22] Sigerist was very clear about that direction: "I do hope I will live long enough to see the triumph of socialism in the world, the beginning of a new era, the promise of civilization at last."[23] Hence, during the Depression and war years, Sigerist, along with other physicians and public health workers, expanded the concern of medical humanism into the political arena.

Controversy was endemic to the medical politics of that period. In the context of the Depression, the issues centered on the access to and organization of medical care. The political left in medicine was struggling for the introduction of national health insurance, government-run clinics, salaried physicians, and pre-paid group practice.[24] What now appear as basic political reforms was seen, in the highly charged atmosphere of the 1930s, as exceedingly radical. Advocates of these positions were often labeled "bolsheviks" and kept from academic appointments.[25]

Sigerist's important role in these efforts was recognized nationally and symbolized by his appearance on the cover of *Time* magazine in 1939, under the lead "His philosophy; history spirals toward socialization."[26] His advocacy of socialized medicine and the Soviet model of health care delivery further identified him as a national spokesman for these causes. Thus Sigerist infused history with a new immediacy. Not surprisingly then, his influence was greatest among an entire generation of physicians enmeshed in medical and health care reforms.[27]

Many of those who considered themselves his students were not formally trained by him at Hopkins, but were touched by his many books, numerous lectures and seminars, and his seemingly boundless energy, friendship, and political support.[28] Milton I. Roemer, now professor of public health at U.C.L.A., recalled that as a young physician in the Public Health Service in Washington, he attended Sigerist's seminars in Baltimore and was encouraged to develop an historical sociological perspective on all his medical policy work.[29] Recounting a meeting of the Medical Advisory Council of the United Automobile Workers in 1943, Sigerist said that what pleased him, "was that everybody congratulated me on my students. Wherever they are, they are doing extremely well. They represent a new type of doctor."[30] The list of some of those influenced by Sigerist spans the political spectrum and reads today like a roll call of many of the leading physicians active in social medicine and public health: Leslie Falk, Ernest Gruenberg, Milton Terris, George Silver, Sy Axelrod, Herbert Abrams, Tom Perry, Cecil Sheps, Lorin Kerr, Hilda Knobloch, Benjamin Pasamanick, Lee Janis, Jonas Muller, Julius Richmond, T. S. Sze, Lester Breslow, Frank Anker, Richard Lippman, Ephraim Kahn, Leonard Rosenfeld, Jeremiah Stamler, and Richard Wienerman.[31]

Sigerist also influenced professional medical historians—among them Ilza Veith, Miriam Drabkin, Genevieve Miller, Owsei Temkin, Erwin Ackerknecht, and George Rosen. But the history of medicine in the 1930s and the 1940s still had a relatively limited institutional base. Chairs and academic appointments were few in number.[32] Even Sigerist's most well-known and prolific intellectual heir, George Rosen, never held an appointment in the history of medicine until he joined the Yale faculty in 1969. Before that, he wrote history while he practiced medicine, worked for the New York City Health Department and the Health Insurance Plan of New York, and taught public health at Columbia.[33]

While Sigerist and his students produced some of the most important work in the history of medicine, they did not represent the dominant approach. The history of medicine remained primarily intellectual history. In addition, both the prevailing political conservatism and the lack of institutional support served to isolate those who were writing left social history. With the rise of McCarthyism in the post-World War II years, the left political import of the social history approach was stifled. Sigerist himself, suffering from ill health, overcommitment, enormous administrative demands, and a growing political uneasiness, left the United States in 1947 to begin writing a synthetic work.[34] He wrote in his diary in 1947:

I did not leave America in order to escape. I left in order to be able
to write my books and made the decision before the situation had
become so acute. When it did become critical I actually thought of
reconsidering my plan, of staying on, waiting for the challenge to
come and of becoming the spokesman for the persecuted left-wing
professors. The alternative was to write my books and to write
articles, to carry on the fight with the pen, to continue my teachings through my books.[35]

The "sociological approach" to medical history was also developed within the discipline of sociology and met with a parallel fate. Bernhard J. Stern, a friend and contemporary of Sigerist's, has been called "the father of medical sociology."[36] His
belief that history provided a framework for understanding
contemporary medical problems is reflected in his pioneering
dissertation on *Social Factors in Medical Progress,* in his books
written for the New York Academy of Medicine, and in his
activities within professional sociology associations.[37] His
clearly articulated Marxist interpretations set medicine within
the contradictions of class conflict without being insensitive to
its peculiarities and its special nature. As an open Marxist,
Stern's academic career at Columbia University, despite his
achievements and skill as a teacher, was precarious. Although
his writing greatly influenced a generation of progressive physicians, his ideas come down to us mainly through his books.
Unlike Sigerist, he had few graduate students and no institute
behind him.[38]

Sigerist, Stern, and their followers, despite their own political
differences, had clearly established that the sociological approach
had much to offer medicine. Although their political views were
at odds with those of the majority of physicians, Sigerist and
Stern were able to make medical history accessible and relevant
to the profession at large. As in the pre-bacteriological era, they
sought to make the history and sociology of medicine an integral part of medical concerns.

The task of integrating social history into the *mainstream* of
medical history was pursued not by a physician but by an historian, Richard H. Shryock, Sigerist's successor in 1949 at the
Hopkins Institute. Shryock brought to medical history a respect
for the social sciences, a commitment to a comparative history

perspective, a sense of the importance of external social forces, and, above all, the sensitivity of a social-cultural historian. His main contribution was to remove medical history from its parochialism and give it a more catholic airing. Shyrock questioned the notion that medicine was always progressing toward truth. He clearly demonstrated that a professional historian, even though not a physician, could write insightfully about medicine's technical aspects.[39] As with others trained in Progressive history, Shryock focused on broad social and cultural currents.[40] Thus for today's social historian his work seems too general, lacking clear explanations of the mechanisms of change.

For intellectual and political reasons, Shryock, unlike Sigerist, was able to start a continuing social history tradition. Sigerist's work was often positivistic and iatrocentric, rooted in an older classical tradition. In contrast, Shryock was able to link medical history to the main currents in the historical profession and "to place medical history in a society-centered cosmos."[41] Their approaches also differed politically. Owsei Temkin summed this up when he noted that there was little hostility toward Shryock because "shorn of political overtones medical sociology was very welcome at Johns Hopkins."[42] Of course Shryock's work did have political overtones, but the tones were not as discordant as Sigerist's in the political and intellectual atmosphere of the 1950s.[43]

Following Shryock, and in conjunction with the post-World War II growth in the field of social history, this approach has slowly become more prominent within the history of medicine.[44] Charles Rosenberg's work is perhaps the clearest example of this. His landmark book, *The Cholera Years,* makes clear that medical history can inform us as much about general social and political change as about science and medicine.[45] Rosenberg symbolizes the conjuncture of medical and general history since he was trained by both types of historians, Erwin H. Ackerknecht and Richard Hofstatder. During the past few years we have seen that the development of social history has been reflected in several collections: Gert Brieger's *Theory and Practice in American Medicine,* Judith Leavitt and Ronald Numbers' *Sickness and Health in America: Readings in the History of Medicine and Public Health,* and a special issue of the *Journal of Social History* devoted to medical history.[46]

Often those writing the social history of medicine today see themselves at the beginning of a new historical tradition. This is in part due to the influx of non-physician historians and to the minority status of the social history impulse within the history of medicine. Many social historians of medicine trace their ancestry to the great English working-class historian, E. P. Thompson, rather than through the intellectual tradition in medical history.[47] The loss of this medical history lineage has import for the future development of the new social history of health care. First, social historians run the risk, as Gerald Grob has noted, of failing to understand the basis for the internal logic of medicine.[48] Second, the sense of urgency and commitment which has fueled much of the important research in medical history may be lost. Social historians of health care are thus in danger of becoming sophisticated antiquarians.

To avoid these pitfalls, social history of health care has to be reinfused with the immediacy which characterized the endeavors of some of its past advocates. We are not trying to suggest that there be what Paul Sanazaro has called "preventive history—drawing on the past to highlight for us potentially undesirable and avoidable consequences of future decisions."[49] Nor do we intend to wrench historical events and forces from their context. Rather, social history can provide an essential tool for analyzing current health care problems by providing a sense both of their origins and the possibilities to affect change. Without this kind of history, the future appears full of chance, inevitability, or irony.

In the preparation of this volume we have incurred many debts. We would like to thank the following people for their assistance: Sam Bloom, Sol Levine, John McKinley, Harry Marks, Charles Rosenberg, and Milton Terris. Our special thanks to Benjamin Pasamanick, Milton Roemer, and Charlotte Stern for taking the time to help bridge the gap between our intellectual generations. Diana Long Hall and Barbara Gutmann Rosenkrantz were always helpful, supportive and, when necessary, critical of this endeavor. Diana Hall's historiographic approach to teaching and her concern with both the art and the science of medicine are two of the intellectual roots of this volume. Barbara Rosenkrantz's insistence on the subtlety and complexity of the historical process and her rigorous standards have given us, as younger scholars, a deep sense of humility. Reuben and

Gertrude Mokotoff have always taught their daughter to respect and value that which is humane and ethical in medicine. Alex and Sophie Rosner have provided their son with a sense of history and its relevance.

As the volume was nearing completion, several people's special efforts made this possible. Kathlyn Conway provided significant technical and editorial assistance. Her critique of various portions of this book was invaluable. Tim Sieber willingly took time away from his own intellectual work to take on more than his share of child care responsibilities and to give the introduction his usual careful reading and criticism. Our editor at Temple University Press, Michael Ames, was always sympathetic and helpful. Donna Scripture retyped our illiterate typing with her usual skill and speed. Finally, in the process of preparing this volume together, we confirmed our belief that the academic enterprise is not intrinsically isolating and that collaborative effort is intellectually rewarding.

Notes

1. Quoted in Erwin H. Ackerknecht, "A Plea for a 'Behaviorist' Approach in Writing the History of Medicine," *Journal of the History of Medicine* 22 (July 1967): 212.
2. Factors internal to the history profession have, of course, affected the development of social history. For a recent discussion of the growth and problems in social history, see *Journal of Social History*, vol. 10 (Winter 1976).
3. For suggestions of the areas to be covered by a social history of medicine and health care, see for examples Gerald Grob, "The Social History of Medicine and Disease in America: Problems and Possibilities," *Journal of Social History* 10 (June 1977): 391-409; Gordon McLachlan and Thomas McKeown, eds., *Medical History and Medical Care* (London: Oxford University Press, 1971); and Richard H. Shryock, "The Historian Looks at Medicine," *Bulletin of the Institute of the History of Medicine* 5 (December 1937): 887-94.
4. Lester King, "Discussion of George Rosen's 'What Medical History Should Be Taught to Medical Students,'" *Education in the History of Medicine*, John B. Blake, ed., Report of Macy Conference, Bethesda, June 22-24, 1966 (New York: Hafner, 1968), p. 45.
5. *The Double Face of Janus* (Baltimore: Johns Hopkins Press, 1977), p. 29.
6. We still do not have a complete social and intellectual study of medical history. Owsei Temkin in his *The Double Face of Janus* has begun this needed exposition. In particular an analysis of the social history impulse, perhaps similar to George Rosen's "What is Social Medicine?" (in

his *From Medical Police to Social Medicine* [New York: Science History Publications, 1974], pp. 60-119) would be an extremely useful beginning.

7. Lloyd Stevenson and Robert Multhauf, eds., *Medicine, Science and Culture: Historical Essays in Honor of Owsei Temkin* (Baltimore: Johns Hopkins Press, 1968), p. xi.

8. Temkin, *Double Face of Janus*, p. 7; George Rosen, "The New History of Medicine," *Journal of the History of Medicine* 6 (Autumn 1951): 516.

9. For discussions of this function of medical history, see Henry R. Viets, *Medical History, Humanism and the Student of Medicine* (Hanover: Dartmouth Press, 1960), and Owsei Temkin, "The Study of the History of Medicine," *Bulletin Johns Hopkins Hospital* 104 (March 1959): 99-106. For a discussion of the modern analog to this, see Guenter B. Risse, "The Role of Medical History in the Education of the 'Humanist' Physician: A Reevaluation," *Journal of Medical Education* 50 (May 1975): 458-65, and Lester S. King et al., "Viewpoints in the Teaching of Medical History," *Clio Medica* 10 (1975): 129-65.

10. "The Binding Influence of a Library on a Subdividing Profession," *Bulletin Johns Hopkins Hospital* 46 (1930): 38.

11. Quoted in Richard H. Shryock, "The Historian Looks at Medicine," *Bulletin of the Institute of the History of Medicine* 5 (December 1937): 887-94.

12. William Osler, "A Note on the Teaching of the History of Medicine," *British Medical Journal* 2 (12 July 1902): 93.

13. "Binding Influence," p. 41.

14. Osler wrote that history was "simply the biography of the mind of man and our interest in history and its educational value to us, is directly proportionate to the completeness of our study of the individual through whom this mind has been manifested." ("Books and Men," *A Way of Life and Selected Writings of Sir William Osler* [New York: Dover Publications, 1958], p. 206).

15. George Rosen, "The Place of History in Medical Education," *Bulletin of the History of Medicine* 22 (September-October 1948): 612-28; see also Erwin Ackerknecht's discussion following Rosen's paper.

16. Ibid.; the problem continued, as Genevieve Miller suggested: "Antiquarianism and mediocre teaching have tended to retard medical history in American medical education, and most medical educators today are unaware of its positive values." ("The Status of Medical History," *Bulletin of the History of Medicine* 43 [May-June 1969]: 267).

17. Genevieve Miller, "The Missing Seal, or Highlights of the First Half Century of the American Association for the History of Medicine," *Bulletin of the History of Medicine* 50 (Spring 1976): 93-115.

18. Nora Sigerist Beeson, ed., *Henry E. Sigerist: Autobiographical Writings* (Montreal: McGill University Press, 1966), p. 64; George Rosen, "Toward a Historical Sociology of Medicine: The Endeavor of Henry E. Sigerist," *Bulletin of the History of Medicine* 32 (November-December 1958): 500-16.

19. Beeson, *Sigerist: Autobiographical Writings*, pp. 216-17.

20. Quoted by Lester King, "Comments," p. 28. For examples, see Milton I. Roemer, ed., *Henry E. Sigerist on the Sociology of Medicine* (New York: MD Publications, 1960); Felix Marti-Ibanez, ed., *Henry E. Sigerist on the History of Medicine* (New York: MD Publications, 1960); George Rosen, "Levels of Integration in Medical Historiography: A Review," *Journal of the History of Medicine* 4 (Autumn 1949): 460-67.

21. For a clear exposition of the tensions Sigerist felt between his classical and political work, see his *Autobiographical Writings.*

22. Ibid., pp. 216-17. Owsei Temkin also discusses Sigerist's views on medical history's "double face"; see Temkin, *Double Face of Janus*, p. 9.

23. Beeson, *Sigerist: Autobiographical Writings*, p. 116.

24. The history of the left in medicine has yet to be written. Lorenzo Finison and Walter Lear are currently working on this topic.

25. Milton I. Roemer, Interview by Susan Reverby, Boston, 21 June 1978.

26. Ibid.; see also Beeson, *Sigerist: Autobiographical Writings*, p. 141.

27. For example, Milton Terris, "The Contributions of Henry E. Sigerist to Health Services Organization," *Milbank Memorial Fund Quarterly/Health and Society,* Fall 1975, pp. 489-530.

28. Benjamin Pasamanick, Interview by David Rosner, Albany, New York, 13 November 1977; see also Beeson, *Sigerist: Autobiographical Writings, passim.*

29. Roemer interview.

30. Beeson, *Sigerist: Autobiographical Writings,* p. 186.

31. This list is by no means complete. Benjamin Pasamanick, Milton I. Roemer, and Milton Terris were extremely helpful in its compilation.

32. Henry Sigerist, "Medical History in the United States," *Bulletin of the History of Medicine* 22 (January-February 1948): 47-63; George Rosen, "The Place of History in Medical Education."

33. Milton Terris, "George Rosen: The Primacy of Ideas," Paper presented at the George Rosen Memorial Seminar, Columbia University, School of Public Health, 17 May 1978.

34. Milton Roemer, "A Tribute to Henry E. Sigerist," *Journal of the History of Medicine* 2 (Autumn 1947): 529-36.

35. Beeson, *Sigerest: Autobiographical Writings*, p. 211.

36. Robert Merton, quoted by Charlotte Stern, Interview by Susan Reverby, New York, 24 June 1978.

37. For examples, see his *Social Factors in Medical Progress,* Columbia Studies in Social Science No. 287, 1927 (New York: AMS edition, 1968); *American Medical Practice* (New York: Commonwealth Fund, 1945); *Medical Services by Government* (New York: Commonwealth Fund, 1946); *Historical Sociology* (New York: Citadel Press, 1959).

38. Milton Terris to Susan Reverby, 15 August 1978.

39. Lloyd G. Stevenson, "A Salute to Richard Shryock," *Journal of the History of Medicine* 23 (January 1968): 7; Merle Curti, "The Historical Scholarship of Richard H. Shryock," *Journal of the History of Medicine* 29 (January 1974): 7-14; Whitfield J. Bell, Jr., "Richard H. Shryock: Life and Work of a Historian," Ibid., pp. 15-31.

40. John Higham, *History: Professional Scholarship in America* (New York: Harper and Row, 1973).

41. Guenter B. Risse, "Introduction, Richard H. Shryock and the Social History of Medicine," *Journal of the History of Medicine* 29 (January 1974): 5. Shryock was told by his dissertation advisor at the University of Pennsylvania that he could not do his thesis on public health; it was "a very good subject, but, of course, it wasn't history" (quoted in *Journal of the History of Medicine* 22 [July 1976] : 322).

42. Temkin, *Double Face of Janus,* p. 29.

43. For a brief discussion of some of the political implications of medical history, see John Burnham, "Will Medical History Join the American Mainstream?" *Reviews in American History* 6 (March 1978): 43-49.

44. For examples of this, see the works of Whitfield Bell, John Blake, John Burnham, James Cassedy, and John Duffy among others.

45. (Chicago: University of Chicago Press, 1962).

46. Gert H. Brieger, ed., *Theory and Practice in American Medicine* (New York: Science History Publications, 1975); Judith Leavitt and Ronald Numbers, eds., *Sickness and Health in America : Readings in the History of Medicine and Public Health* (Madison: University of Wisconsin Press, 1978); *Journal of Social History* vol. 10 (June 1977). A new Marxist historiography is developing; see Howard S. Berliner, "Philanthropic Foundations and Scientific Medicine," (Ph.D. diss., Department of Medical Care and Hospitals, Johns Hopkins University, 1977); Linda Gordon, *Women's Body, Women's Right: A Social History of Birth Control in America* (New York: Grossman, 1976); *Health Movement Organization,* Packet no. 1 (Washington, D.C.: Political Economy Program Center, Institute for Policy Studies, 1976). pp. 4-7.

47. Thompson's major work is *The Making of the English Working Class* (New York: Vintage, 1963). Charles Rosenberg brought this point to our attention.

48. "The Social History of Medicine and Disease in America."

49. "Historical Discontinuity, Hospitals and Health Services," *Medical History and Medical Care,* Gordon McLachlan and Thomas McKeown, eds. (London: Oxford University Press, 1971), p. 131.

PART II

THE PUBLIC, PHYSICIANS, AND POLITICIANS: THE SHIFTING BOUNDARIES OF MEDICAL CARE

In recent years consumer groups have challenged professional dominance over the definitions of health, disease, and the provision of health services. Underlying these challenges are historical questions concerning the shifting boundaries between professional and lay control. The following four articles address changing views on who should control these definitions and practices.

The selection by Lawrence G. Miller explores the introduction of a particular technique of anesthesia, the twilight sleep, in childbirth and the conflict between women and the medical profession over its use. He investigates the definition of childbirth as a pathological process and concludes that such a definition was a product of the politics and social role of medicine as much as a result of the perceived biological reality of parturition.

Martha Verbrugge looks at the manner in which middle-class women sought to gain knowledge about personal health in nineteenth-century America. Verbrugge suggests that health became a focus for them when social relationships within the family and the very economic and social functions of the family changed. She posits that concern with health grew as other aspects of life became uncertain.

Virginia G. Drachman looks at a particular innovation in medical education and the resultant popular and professional reaction to it. She illustrates the intertwining relationship between lay and professional attitudes as well as the major differences which separated medical educators, generalists, and the lay public in nineteenth-century America.

Judith Walzer Leavitt investigates the political consequences of differences in medical opinion. Her work is a study of political and community responses to public health measures—specifically, the case of a smallpox hospital in an immigrant working class neighborhood.

These articles all address a central issue: the complex relationship between medicine and social control. How do medical and technological innovations reflect underlying class and political differences? The articles also raise questions about class, sex, and ethnic-specific responses to public health and medical measures. How do different groups organize to meet their health needs, and how does medicine respond to consumer demands?

LAWRENCE G. MILLER

2 Pain, Parturition, and the Profession: Twilight Sleep in America

As symbol, childbirth reflects and helps shape societal views of women's nature. Nowhere is this more explicit than in the biblical curse placed on Eve: "I will greatly multiply thy sorrow and thy conception: in sorrow thou shalt bring forth children."[1] Not only did childbirth become symbolic of woman's transgression, but the pain of childbirth was thus explained and justified. In our society the relationship between physicians and women, and the extent to which physicians become involved in the birth process, depends not only on the notion of childbirth but also on what is understood as the duty of the physician with regard to pain and disease. In the early twentieth century these issues were reflected in the controversy about "twilight sleep," then a new form of obstetric anesthesia.

The introduction of anesthesia into obstetrics in 1847 encountered stiff opposition on religious and medical grounds. Within the next few decades, however, resistance in the form of attacks on anesthesia declined.[2] Still, many births, probably about one-half, were supervised by midwives who had little knowledge of anesthesia.[3] Of those births that occurred in hospitals, few were accompanied by anesthesia.[4] The use of anesthesia in home births attended by physicians is more difficult to assess. General practitioners, with little inclination to read or write in medical journals, performed the great majority of medical deliveries.[5] Nonetheless, the occasional appearance of papers in medical journals exhorting practitioners to employ obstetric

I would like to thank Ms. L. J. Daston for her criticism. I am indebted to the staffs of Countway Library and Schlessinger Library for their assistance.

19

anesthetics suggests the rarity of the technique. As late as 1894 one writer chastised his colleagues for continuing to stand by "wakefully and helplessly," arguing that the duty of the obstetrician included "preventing or banishing birth pain."[6] Similar points of view were presented in obstetric textbooks, and in popular medical manuals written by physicians.[7] Anesthesia was in use, but in a minority of cases.

The twilight sleep consisted of the drugs morphine and scopolamine. The combination was first applied to obstetrics in 1902 by Von Steinbuchel in Graz, Germany, and was extended by C. J. Gauss in Freiburg.[8] As practiced in Freiburg, it consisted of repeated small injections of scopolamine and morphine beginning soon after cervical dilatation. The level of anesthesia was monitored by a memory test given several times an hour: If the patient could not remember series of numbers, anesthesia was deemed sufficient. As such, twilight sleep constituted amnesia and analgesia rather than true anesthesia. As a contemporary observer noted, the patient "gives every outward evidence during her confinement of acute suffering. She cries out as others do under suffering; tells the doctor perhaps that her pains are severe beyond endurance." But after the delivery is complete and the child is presented to her, "she does not recognize the child as her own, or realize that she has yet been delivered." To protect the amnesic state, efforts were made to reduce stimuli impinging on the mother: a darkened room, dark glasses, ear plugs, quiet staff. Otherwise, "memory islands," brief vignettes of pain, might remain after delivery. Gauss claimed success, complete amnesia, in 80 percent of his patients, and further cited the advantage of having the "conscious" patient aid the physician in the childbirth process.[9]

In the meantime, the Freiburg experience stimulated experimentation with twilight sleep in Britain, France, and the United States.[10] Charles M. Green, a professor of obstetrics at Harvard, was one of the first to use scopolamine-morphine in 1906, but he soon gave up because of poor results.[11] F. S. Newell, also at Harvard, reported considerably more success with 41 cases in 1906.[12] In 1907 he reported 127 further cases of twilight sleep and concluded that scopolamine-morphine was "an efficient means of controlling the pain of labor".[13] Others were even more enthusiastic—one called scopolamine-morphine the "ideal anesthetic" that would banish the "exhausting ordeal of mother-hood."[14]

Others were far less sanguine. Some gave the technique only a short trial, while others reported that "bad results and deaths were numerous."[15] It should be noted that none of the American obstetricians, whether successful or not, followed the Freiburg method in detail. Most used larger doses, employing the memory test only rarely, which may account for the mixed results. Still, the number of favorable reports was sufficient to prompt De Lee, a well-known obstetrician, to publish a request for "bad results," since most accounts had been favorable.[16] The method received little attention in medical journals, and the conclusions in a major 1912 textbook probably represented the prevailing opinion: Scopolamine-morphine prolonged labor and asphyxiated infants.[17] Twilight sleep received even less notice in the lay press. One maternity manual of 1907 mentioned the technique, but only to speculate that it was excessively dangerous.[18]

Interest in the twilight sleep was revived in 1913 by a visit from Bernhard Kronig of Freiburg clinic. Although invited to speak before the Clinical Conference of Surgeons on the use of radium in gynecologic diseases, he spent much of his time discussing twilight sleep. He reiterated his justification for anesthesia in labor, cited the success of twilight sleep at Freiburg, and concluded that "the decreasing capacity for resisting pain shown by cultured, civilized women seems to us urgently to call for measures which can reduce the pains of childbirth."[19] Kronig's talk prompted lively discussion but little other apparent professional response. However, *McClure's* magazine, sensing a story of intense public interest, commissioned journalists Marguerite Tracy and Mary Boyd to travel to Freiburg and investigate twilight sleep. Mrs. Boyd was also to undergo twilight sleep for the birth of her expected child.[20]

Few American women were familiar with the twilight sleep or Freiburg until the publication of the first article in *McClure's* of June 1914, entitled "Painless Childbirth." In this article Marguerite Tracy and Constance Leupp described the "new and painless method of childbirth," exulting that "modern science has abolished that primal sentence of the Scriptures upon womankind." They reported twilight sleep to be safe for mother and child, cited the theory that civilization had rendered women unfit to endure pain, and quoted at length from the papers of Gauss and Kronig. Criticisms of twilight sleep were attributed to improper technique, especially in large hospitals where the method would not be properly employed.[21]

The *McClure's* article generated a tremendous popular response; a sequel, published in October, reported that: "No article ever published in *McClure's* attracted more attention than 'Painless Childbirth,' in the June issue."[22] This article chastised obstetricians for not embracing painless childbirth, comparing childbirth to a surgical procedure. It was even implied that twilight sleep children were healthier than their conventionally delivered siblings. Other articles soon appeared in women's magazines: *Ladies World,* claiming a circulation of one million, published a description of Mrs. Boyd's experience at Freiburg and appended a section suggesting that American women demand painless childbirth, forcing the cooperation of their physicians if necessary.[23] The *Woman's Home Companion* of January 1915 discussed a theme often repeated in letters to the "Expectant Mother's Circle": "Tell me, please, the truth about the Twilight Sleep; is it practical; is it available; is it safe—for me?"[24] In 1915 the *Literary Digest* summarized the first stage of twilight sleep publicity: "There can be no doubt that it was the most widely known and most generally talked about medical achievement of last year."[25]

While limited popular response was essentially enthusiastic, the response of the American medical profession to the wave of twilight sleep publicity was scathing. During the next few months the medical controversy revolved around three major issues: lay agitation for twilight sleep and its perceived commercial overtones; the relief of pain in childbirth; and the merits of the twilight sleep itself. Early medical critics expressed outrage at the lay interference in a medical matter. A typical editorial in the *Journal of the American Medical Association* labeled the *McClure's* article as "pseudoscientific rubbish" and railed against "this shameless exploitation of the fears of the prospective mothers of the country."[26] Although a few applauded the revived interest in obstetrics due to twilight sleep agitation, even proponents of the method acknowledged the deleterious effects of lay publicity; one physician reported that lay publicity had created a "strong prejudice against the twilight sleep within the medical profession."[27]

To other medical critics, the twilight sleep publicity "savored strongly of commercialism." Another physician called it "quackish hocus-pocus advocated by our notoriety seeking German contemporaries."[28] While this represents an extreme position, *Modern Hospital* perceived a consensus that "Kronig and Gauss overstepped the bounds of professional propriety in advertising themselves," especially soon after Kronig's Chicago appearance.[29]

Its foreign origin served as yet another argument for those who rejected twilight sleep, seeking instead to "relieve the modern American mother by modern American methods."[30] Whether favorable or not, the publicity and popular response to twilight sleep made the issue of painless childbirth an important one.[31]

Women in Milwaukee responded to the negative views of physicians by condemning the local medical society.[32] (This response illustrates the strength of popular support for twilight sleep and the reasons underlying medical outrage at lay agitation.) Many supporters of twilight sleep were, indeed, indicting the medical profession for its failure to attend to painless childbirth and for its refusal to consider this new technique.[33] Even medical proponents such as Harrar and McPherson wondered why "detailed descriptions of the technic [sic] . . . have lain idle in the literature for 6 years with no one taking advantage of them."[34]

The adversary nature of the controversy was explicitly recognized. Some urged women to study twilight sleep so as to avoid "having to ask questions of their doctors." Others questioned the "doctor's discretion"—"administration of painlessness shall not be left to the decision of the doctor, but to the mother." The twilight sleep was hailed as a movement: "It is, as far as we know, the first time in the history of medical science that the whole body of patients have risen to dictate to the doctors."[35]

In addition, the scornful medical response brought a barrage of rebuttals from twilight sleep advocates and the lay press. Carter, a twilight sleep popularizer, blamed the AMA monopoly for medical intransigence.[36] Throughout the fall of 1914 and the spring of 1915, the *New York Times* constantly sniped at the medical profession from its editorial page. Early on, the *Times* predicted that medical authority would be defeated and criticized arguments against twilight sleep as premature, irrelevant, and even deliberately distorted.[37] It was noted sarcastically that the tendency of male physicians was to view the "torture" of labor with a "beautiful calm."[38] Other newspapers, while less opinionated, nevertheless repeated the themes of professional obstinancy and conservatism.[39]

Despite the vigor of the controversy, the disagreement between supporters and detractors of twilight sleep rested upon an underlying consensus as to the importance of childbirth and the role of physicians in its conduct. By 1914 feminist agitation for suffrage and women's rights had become widespread and vocal.[40] A few critics suggested that feminists had rejected motherhood along with submissiveness.[41] This view, however, is supported neither by feminist literature nor by the writings of twilight sleep proponents. In feminist writings Ellen Key, an inspiration to "the woman movement," described motherhood as the natural function of women.[42] Physicians and twilight sleep advocates such as Tracy and Boyd concurred: Motherhood was the "sublime primal function of Mother Earth."[43] Neither did advocates of twilight sleep question the physician's ultimate control of the childbirth process, despite their demands for twilight sleep. To Tracy and Boyd, childbirth was potentially a "great emergency," and the relief of suffering in childbirth not only was humane but also transformed parturition "from a gross and primitive physical agony to a normal unimpeded muscular process which can be entirely directed by the obstetrician."[44]

Physicians explicitly recognized the importance of control and the use of anesthesia in maintaining that control. A major advantage of anesthesia, as one physician claimed, was that it gave "absolute control over your patient at all stages of the game. . . . You are 'boss'."[45] While these physicians clearly intended to emphasize control over technical aspects of labor, the importance attached to the dominance of the physician is implicit. The position was made explicit by Newell: "My object in taking care of an obstetric case is to leave as little as possible to every parturient woman as a doubtful risk medically."[46]

The agitation for medical control of childbirth reflects the tenuous position of the early twentieth-century American physician, and the obstetrician in particular. The physician felt the pressure of competition acutely, for the profession was widely believed to be overcrowded.[47] In addition, folk healers, patent medicine, Christian Science, or "New Thought" also threatened to lure away the physician's source of income.[48] To obstetricians, childbirth was only then becoming viewed as a problem requiring medical expertise. To survive, an obstetrician had to make himself or herself indispensable. Thus, he or she had to demonstrate complete control of the childbirth process and technological measures could serve to augment this control.[49]

The twilight sleep controversy thus reaffirmed the maternal role of women and the importance of childbirth. It further affirmed the dominance of the physician during parturition. The latter was achieved, as Newell illustrates, by the definition of labor as pathological.

Whether labor was physiological or pathological in character has been long debated, especially with reference to the necessity of pain. Benjamin Rush, the early nineteenth-century physician, for example, thought that childbearing was a disease and that pain could be eliminated.[50] Similar arguments were propounded by early advocates of obstetrical anesthesia, but the issue was by no means resolved in 1914. Two general positions were presented: Labor was physiological and therefore pain was natural, even helpful; and the pain of labor rendered the process pathological by definition. Those who maintained the value of pain were in the minority in medical journals but may have represented the majority of practitioners. They presented three major arguments: Pain was physiological, pain excited maternal love, and pain aided the practitioner. *American Medicine* editorialized that complaints about pain often came from "hysterical and nervous women" and pains caused no "discoverable bad result."[51] One author quoted a physician who advanced the second argument: "I believe that women should bring forth in pain and suffering for thereby her appreciation and love of her child is increased."[52] Others cited the value of pain in "guiding" the obstetrical forceps.[53]

These arguments were rejected by physicians committed to the relief of labor pains. They accepted the pains as genuine and contended that such pain was excessive for a truly physiological event. Further, they sought to explain the pathological origin of pain. Religious justifications for pain were dismissed as "amusing," although their effect was probably still felt.[54] Some sought an anatomical rationale to reject the necessity of pain.[55] Williams, a Hopkins obstetrician concerned with reforming the specialty, described the contradictory nature of pain: From an evolutionary standpoint pain was adaptive in preserving the individual, but in discouraging childbearing it was "positively menacing to the race." A truly natural process would be painless, so pain was paradoxical: "Natural labor is an easy, short, painless act."[56]

But if natural labor were painless, why did twentieth-century labor involve pain? An obvious resolution was achieved: That modern labor was unnatural. This conclusion was supported by a wealth of anthropological evidence garnered from the late nineteenth-century interest in primitives. One author maintained that their labor was "short and easy, accompanied by few accidents and followed by little or no prostration."[57] Popular manuals cited similar evidence and included the robust women of the poorer classes with the primitives.[58] Such evidence led to the conclusion that labor pains are "an extraneous and in a sense abnormal product of civilization."[59]

Two particular aspects of civilization were held responsible for pains in childbirth: Unnatural customs and a sensitive nervous system. To one author, women had become a "hot-house product" due to customs such as "tight lacing (of corsets) and insufficient physical culture." Civilization had further rendered the nervous systems of the "upper highly civilized class of woman" acutely sensitive and thus unable to bear the "shock" of childbirth. To some, this process had been exacerbated by the education of women. Pain was the inevitable accompaniment of the progress of civilization.[60]

The evils of pain and the benefits to be derived from relieving pain were clear to the advocates of anesthesia. Some posited that painful impulses were carried through the nervous system to the brain, where brain cell exhaustion and deterioration occurred. Thus, excessive pain could cause shock or even lasting mental deterioration. The accompanying exhaustion slowed a mother's recovery and left her less well fit to care for her child.[61] In addition, pain in childbirth was said to lengthen labor and to predispose the mother to lacerations and forceps deliveries. Accordingly, the relief of pain would render labor safer, banish nervous exhaustion, result in healthier mothers

and healthier offspring, and, by eliminating the fear of childbirth, would ensure the development of proper mental attitudes during pregnancy.[62] It was contended that anesthesia
would once again make childbirth natural: The control of labor
would return to "the reflex ganglia from which the brain had
. . . taken it away."[63] Pain was thus normal but unnatural;
what was "natural" had been redefined by twilight sleep advocates to include the use of anesthesia.

A basic agreement again underlies the controversy over twilight sleep, both sides assumed the efficacy of medicine to treat
parturition. The major area of contention was not whether to
relieve pain in labor but rather which method to use. Many obstetricians violently opposed twilight sleep but accepted the use
of other anesthetics in childbirth.

The arguments concerning twilight sleep were broad-ranging
and sophisticated, from the use of twilight sleep in the home to
subtle issues of dosage and technique.[64] First, opponents of the
technique frequently cited their own experience as unfavorable.
De Lee, for example, writing soon after the original *McClure's*
article, reported that he and others had used the method some
years previously with unsatisfactory results. A second major
type of criticism involved the practical problems with the
method and its resulting limited utility. Even proponents of twilight sleep suggested that it be confined to hospitals, and there
to the private service.[65] The general practitioner was thus excluded from using twilight sleep. The time required by the
method was thought to limit its appeal among obstetricians as
well. The concomitant expense and the better results with
upper-class women were also cited as restricting its use.[66]

Medical proponents of the twilight sleep anticipated a few
of these arguments and attempted to refute others. Williams, for
example, stressed the necessity of adhering to the Freiburg
method, warning that deviation might cause harm and discredit
the twilight sleep in general. Another attacked the "absurd
claims" made by twilight sleep opponents, especially the association with insanity. Still others claimed that twilight sleep
resulted in a shortened first stage of labor, lower infant mortality, fewer operative deliveries, and absence of postpartum exhaustion.[67] Few obstetricians viewed the twilight sleep as a
panacea; almost all qualified their praise by pointing out the
necessity of carefully controlled conditions and trained per-

sonnel.[68] In this respect many twilight sleep advocates agreed with their opposition: The method was not universally applicable at present, and it was emphatically the method of the obstetrician rather than the general practitioner.[69]

Finally, proponents of twilight sleep claimed the method had eugenic advantages.[70] Twilight sleep advocates attributed the declining birthrate among the better "classes" at least partially to the fear of labor pains. They emphasized in particular the applicability of the technique to the cultured woman with the "higher type of intellect"; these women would "have more babies if they know they can have them without pain."[71]

Lay supporters of twilight sleep presented similar arguments, albeit with fewer reservations.[72] It was agreed that twilight sleep would remove the fear of childbirth and therefore increase the fecundity of the race. Publicists also joined obstetricians in warning of the dangers of the alternative scopolamine and morphine methods, and in emphasizing the need for trained accoucheurs. While the general practitioner was criticized for his or her poor training and lack of expertise, Tracy and Boyd hoped that the detailed description of the Freiburg technique would enable both obstetrician and general practitioner alike to use twilight sleep.[73] Other writers emphasized the return to "natural" labor promoted by the method; the decreased strain on the mother, leaving her "physical powers conserved," promised a "new era" for women.[74]

Not only did twilight sleep promise a new era for women, but a new era for obstetrics as well. Accordingly, some obstetricians promoted the twilight sleep as an instrument for the reform of obstetrics. Knipe and Polak, for instance, held that twilight sleep would lead to more careful, scientific obstetrics.[75] A recurrent theme pervaded the writings of those who sought obstetric reform; obstetrics must be made comparable to its more respected colleague, surgery. Knipe reminded his readers that in surgery "infinite care" was taken to relieve pain; Polak compared the expertise required by the obstetrician to that of the surgeon. He went on to suggest that painless obstetrics, like surgery, would be safer in hospitals.[76]

Obstetrics in the early twentieth century had just begun the arduous process of professionalization.[77] The first obstetrical societies began to meet in the latter part of the nineteenth century, and the first maternity hospitals were erected at this time.

The Section on Obstetrics and Gynecology of the American Medical Association was not created until 1903. To many obstetricians of the period, the field had not yet attained the status of a medical specialty. Midwives attended about one-half of urban childbirths, perhaps more in rural areas; general practitioners attended most of the others; and obstetricians only a few.[78] Several authors also cited the lack of improvement in mortality statistics as evidence of the need for reform, while others decried the "gross lesions" frequently sustained in childbirth.[79] A movement to reform obstetrics was championed by J. W. Williams, professor at Johns Hopkins. His plans included regulation of medical schools, abolition of midwives, strict licensing regulation, and construction of hospital maternity facilities. He had the support of many obstetricians, regardless of their affiliation with twilight sleep.[80]

Lay advocates of twilight sleep cited similar arguments.[81] They emphasized, however, the importance of twilight sleep; improvement in obstetrics was merely serendipitous. Leupp and Hendrick, for example, envisioned a *Dammerschlaf* hospital, where "science, surgical dexterity, and painlessness will prevail."[82]

Again, many participants in the twilight sleep controversy shared the assumption that obstetrics was in need of reform. At issue was the place of twilight sleep in that reform. To some obstetricians the prime goal was the reform of obstetrics; twilight sleep was important but ultimately incidental. Lay publicists usually saw the issue in a different light; twilight sleep was the essential reform and obstetrical improvement a by-product. The same innovation thus fueled two distinct but overlapping reform movements.

By early 1915 twilight sleep reformers had reason to celebrate. As Carter put it, opposition seemed to be "rapidly giving way."[83] By November 1914 five hospitals in New York had delivered one thousand women without accident.[84] In February 1915 the number of hospitals using twilight sleep was steadily increasing "in response to an irresistable demand by women."[85]

Physicians also seemed to be moderating their original opposition. In January 1915 the twilight sleep was hailed at the meeting of the Chicago Medical Society with little opposition, and a similar event occurred at the AMA meeting in San Francisco a few months later.[86] Leupp and Hendrick related a different measure of the success of the technique: The "hotel corridors of Freiburg are fairly jammed with medical men from this country."[87]

Another index of medical acceptance can be found in two surveys. Anna Steese Richardson, for *McClure's* magazine, sampled major American cities, finding the greatest twilight sleep agitation in New York and increasing acceptance on the West Coast and in the Midwest.[88] Hellman sent questionnaires to all fellows of the American College of Surgery who had expressed interest in obstetrics. Of the forty who replied, twenty-six had tried twilight sleep and twenty-one planned to continue using the method.[89]

The extent of twilight sleep support among women is more difficult to estimate since few records remain. Nevertheless, some direct and much indirect evidence allows inferences to be made. Tracy and Boyd claimed that four to five million women were involved in the twilight sleep movement. They stressed the importance of widespread participation, including the "ordinary women who does not belong to clubs."[90] Davis, an obstetrician and twilight sleep critic, appears to have been more accurate; despite efforts to involve all classes of women, the major interest and support came from clubwomen.[91]

In the early twentieth century women's clubs formed a powerful, self-described "movement" with a characteristic participant: the "clubwoman."[92] Such women proudly embraced traditional values: The child's place was at the mother's knee, and the mother's place was in the home. Still, a woman's task went far beyond childrearing to include the preservation and improvement of the race. Clubwomen were concerned with suffrage, factory conditions for women workers, women's education for community service, prostitution, child labor, and treatment of servants. While the issues affected all segments of society, the composition and direction of the movement was decidedly middle- to upper-class.

The issue of twilight sleep was ideally suited to these women. It had been publicized in journals appealing to them, such as *McClure's* and *Ladies Home Journal.* Clubwomen also had the time, interest, and means to consult obstetricians. Further, twilight sleep had been presented as particularly suited to the nervous systems of women of the upper classes. It was not surprising, then, that of the "tremendous number of women" discussing the Freiburg method, it had become an especially "vital topic of discussion at women's clubs and gatherings."[93] A group of New York clubwomen, spurred by such discussions, founded the National Twilight Sleep Association (NTSA) in early 1915.[94]

The NTSA was emphatically a clubwomen's organization. All members of its executive committee were "society" women, and eight of twenty were listed in *Who's Who Among American Women* for 1914-1915. The committee included several prominent members of the National American Woman's Suffrage Association, and the NTSA was soon endorsed by the New York Federation of Women's Clubs. The NTSA had three major goals: To sponsor a lecture series publicizing the technique, to circulate pamphlets advocating the twilight sleep, and to agitate for a teaching hospital designed specifically for twilight sleep. A series of talks was held in department stores and theatres in major eastern cities; speakers included obstetricians who were advocates of twilight sleep, such as John O. Polak and Eliza Taylor Ransom, and, almost invariably, mothers who had undergone twilight sleep exhibited their children.[95] Boston newspapers reported that hundreds were turned away from crowded department stores during these twilight sleep talks.[96] Pamphlets, such as a reprint of an address by obstetrician W. H. W. Knipe, were printed and widely distributed through these meetings.[97] Efforts toward the third goal, a twilight sleep hospital, were initiated in early 1915 by a group of women associated with the Caledonian Hospital in Brooklyn, led by Mrs. Francis X. Carmody.[98]

After the first wave of twilight sleep publicity in 1914, Eliza Taylor Ransom, a woman physician and clubwoman, became an active twilight sleep proponent. She studied the method at the Massachusetts Homeopathic Hospital, among the first institutions to experiment with twilight sleep. In November 1914 she opened the Twilight Sleep Maternity Hospital in a well-to-do area of Boston. The thirty-bed hospital was advertised as "A Thoroughly-equipped Modern Maternity House" away from the "Commotion, Noise, Hustle, and Responsibility of one's own Home or the General Hospital." Twilight sleep and other anesthetics were employed; graduate nurses in residence, and outside physicians could deliver their own cases.[99] The hospital was by no means a charity; its rates were at least that of other Boston hospitals.[100] Boston newspapers soon reported that the well-to-do were patronizing the Twilight Sleep Hospital, and by mid-1915 Ransom reported that the twilight sleep was being espoused by Boston society women.[101]

In addition to her obstetric efforts, Ransom also spoke at various twilight sleep meetings, including women's clubs and a mass meeting attended by a "big Audience of stylish women."[102] Her articles advocating twilight sleep appeared in medical journals, newspapers, and clubwomen's publications. Ransom emphasized themes common to most twilight sleep proponents: The inutility of pain, the safety of the method, the importance of improving the race, and the contribution to the obstetric reform.[103]

Ransom's career, while bridging the gap between obstetric and lay advocates of twilight sleep, nevertheless illustrates several important characteristics of twilight sleep supporters: Their upper social class origin, their club affiliation, and their allegiance to other philanthropic or reform movements. The suffrage movement was most obviously associated with twilight sleep, as illustrated by the prominence in suffrage activities of members of NTSA. Ransom pointed out the connection between the two movements: Twilight sleep could enable a woman to become " a more useful and democratic member of society."[104] Other twilight sleep supporters, both lay and medical, were more explicit. Wakefield, an obstetrician, equated the "right to bear children without suffering untold anguish" with other women's rights efforts.[105]

The twilight sleep movement was not an isolated medical crusade supplemented by a few lay publicists, but rather a reform movement situated within the network of other progressive reforms. Several themes common to progressive reform movements can be abstracted: Middle class origins, interest in efficiency, faith in scientific progress, and an emphasis on the child.[106] The twilight sleep movement, to a greater or lesser degree, embodied each of these themes, especially those of science and the child. Civilization had made childbearing unnatural, interfering with the crucial function of motherhood. The answer was not, of course, to question civilization; progressive reforms looked not backward but forward. A new order could be created solving traditional problems, and the twilight sleep was part of that new order.

From its zenith in early 1915, the twilight sleep movement plummeted rapidly and was moribund by the end of the year. Continued professional opposition and a crucial misfortune were responsible for this sudden demise. By early 1915 the professional opposition that had appeared to be waning had surfaced anew. Resentment of lay intrusion into medical affairs and continued association with commercialism fired many protests. *American Medicine,* upon learning of the formation of the NTSA, wondered whether its members were the "same people who are opposed to vaccination and vivisection." It was certain that physicians "will not be stampeded by these misguided ladies."[107] Other journals voiced similar opinions—medical questions were for medical experts to decide.

To some extent, twilight sleep publicity proved counterproductive, as predicted by several proponents. The rush to adopt the method often resulted in poor adherence to the Freiburg technique, with concomitant morbidity and mortality. In February 1915, under the title, "Safeguarding Against Scopolamine Casualties," the Michael Reese Hospital in Chicago announced that it would not use twilight sleep without a waiver of liability from the patient.[108] Amidst considerable publicity, other hospitals in New York, Philadelphia, Cleveland, and elsewhere soon followed suit.[109] By early August the most prestigious institution in the country, Johns Hopkins, announced abandonment of the technique.[110] To be sure, these were all city hospitals serving largely charity patients, and some twilight sleep proponents had doubted the applicability of the method to these hospitals. Nonetheless, the publicity attendant to these rejections of twilight sleep discouraged both physicians and mothers from using the technique.[111]

The NTSA recognized the ill effects of such publicity and attempted to counter it by holding a meeting in New York in April 1915. In calling the meeting, the sponsors cited "the report that certain local hospitals have dropped twilight sleep" and claimed that this attack demanded a "vigorous reply."[112] One hundred and fifty society women were present to hear both Polak and Ransom speak on the problems created by improper technique in twilight sleep administration. Ransom went so far as to propose a federal law forbidding the use of twilight sleep without special training.[113]

The meeting drew considerable publicity but an even more severe blow was dealt the twilight sleep movement in August 1915 with the death of Mrs. Francis X. Carmody. Among the first women to travel to Freiburg to obtain twilight sleep, Mrs. Carmody then became a prominent member of the NTSA's executive committee. Her death during a twilight sleep childbirth received extensive publicity, causing irreparable harm to the movement. Despite protestations that "the twilight sleep treatment was not involved" in her death, the incident appeared to confirm the worst predictions of twilight sleep opponents.[114] Soon after, a friend and neighbor of Carmody initiated an anti-twilight sleep movement to alert well-to-do women to the dangers of the technique.[115]

The day after Carmody's death the *New York Times* announced that twilight sleep was dead.[116] Without referring specifically to the incident the preceding day, the editorial cited widespread publicity surrounding the dangers of twilight sleep and its rejection by various hospitals: "The attempt to create a general and insistent demand by women for relief has been, for the present, defeated."[117] Although some advocates of twilight sleep, such as Knipe and Ransom, continued their efforts, the NTSA soon disintegrated. The failure of the twilight sleep was not difficult for its advocates to explain. Three reasons were frequently cited for its lack of success: German origin; adverse publicity, especially that of rejection by the Johns Hopkins Hospital, and the difficulty of the method for the general practitioner.[118]

A more subtle rationale for the failure of twilight sleep was advanced by a physician, Bertha Van Hoosen. Writing somewhat later and in retrospect, she ascribed the problem partially to the control of the process of parturition: "The obstetrical patient is quite at the mercy of the attending physician in every respect, but especially in regard to anesthesia." Until a woman gained footing similar to the obstetrician's, the process would be his rather than hers, and the decision to use anesthesia would be made accordingly.[119]

Perhaps the most compelling explanation was that of a Doctor Aranow, who wrote "A Post-Mortem on Twilight Sleep" in

1918. He queried:

> What is wrong with twilight sleep? What has happened to the en-
> thusiasts who hailed it as the greatest discovery since Mother Eve
> tasted the forbidden fruit? Why have the men who have proclaimed
> the wonders of the twilight sleep suddenly grown mute? Why has it
> gone into practical oblivion after such a short life?[120]

His answer was simple: "My opinion is that twilight sleep died a
sudden death, not through lack of real merit, but because it
failed to live up to a false reputation."[121] To Aranow, twilight
sleep advocates, both physicians and patients, expected too
much. Physicians were led to expect a method that would substantially reduce the problems and complications of childbirth.
Instead, they found a technique that required constant vigilance
and depended on a subjective memory test. Lay reformers, who
looked to the twilight sleep to solve many of the problems of
motherhood, even of women in general, discovered that the twilight sleep was not a panacea for those ills. They seriously under-
estimated other influences on women's roles and health.

Further, widespread dissemination of the twilight sleep movement was precluded by the nature of the method. The huge
majority of women were delivered by midwives or general practitioners, for whom the method was unavailable or impractical.
In addition, relatively few births took place in hospitals, except
among the poor. The rest occurred in homes, where twilight
sleep was acknowledged to be difficult. Without sweeping social
change, twilight sleep could have had only limited utility.

Finally, a similar argument applies to the twilight sleep movement itself. Despite the enthusiastic efforts of the NTSA, it
remained a relatively localized, class-specific movement. The
"average" women envisioned by Tracy and Boyd did not materialize; instead, organized agitation remained confined to clubwomen, mainly in the Northeast. Clubwomen's reforms had succeeded in the past. But arrayed in opposition to the twilight
sleep was the defensive, even hostile, medical profession, whose
somewhat precarious position was obviously threatened by lay
intrusion into medical affairs. As Van Hoosen pointed out, the
physician retained control of the birth process. Only a massive
movement, and one with different assumptions than the twilight sleep movement, could have succeeded in weakening this
control.

Although twilight sleep advocates failed to achieve their grandiose goals, the controversy served to crystallize many of the unarticulated ideas that had been brought to consensus over the previous several decades. First, childbirth came to be viewed as a pathological rather than a physiological condition.[122] Perhaps the clearest statement of this was made by a Dr. Brant, writing soon after the controversy in 1916: "Pregnancy has not inaptly been called a disease of nine months' duration. We might add that the disease is always terminated by a surgical procedure, namely labor."[123] Brant naturally drew practice from theory: Childbirth was a disease, and medical intervention was therefore justified, even necessary.

Subsequent authors accepted this premise and logic. To Raiford, addressing himself to the general practitioner in 1923, a new type of obstetric work was necessary:

> The intense interest manifested in recent years by all prospective mothers in twilight sleep and other forms of pain relieving methods as advocated or used during childbirth forces us to realize the absolute necessity of abandoning the old "watchful waiting" method of handling our obstetric work and adopting in its stead an "up and doing" policy in these cases.[124]

Raiford cited such intervention as a hallmark of modern obstetrics. He noted a "striking" shift in the past ten years, from "allowing nature to take its course" to "correcting abnormal conditions."[125] Childbirth had become a medical problem, and the control, direction, and intervention into the childbirth process was a medical responsibility.

The second theme to emerge from the twilight sleep controversy was the duty of the obstetrician to relieve labor pains, the most important of the "abnormal conditions." Kostmayer in 1916 recalled his early obstetrical training in which pain was taught as "necessary and natural." However, the situation had changed: "The women themselves have forced on us the problem of relieving, or at least minimizing their pain, and the problem must be resolved if the profession is to do its duty toward womankind."[126] By 1923 Danforth and Davis could confidently conclude that "there can be no controversy at the present time as to the desirability of relief of pain in labor."[127]

In practice the efforts to relieve pain often included the twilight sleep or a modified version thereof. Hence the third theme of the twilight sleep legacy: the limited acceptance of the method itself. While discussing the failure of the twilight sleep movement, Aranow concluded that "scopolamine and morphine nevertheless have a distinct and merited place in the practice of obstetrics."[128] Wakefield[129] in 1918, and Schwartz[130] in 1919 defined such a niche as the first stage of labor. By 1923 De Normandie could report: "I never hesitate to use morphia and chloral [hydrate] and scopolamine to take [women] over this trying [first] stage."[131] Others concurred.The twilight sleep had become part of the obstetrician's armamentarium.

The fourth and final theme inherent in the twilight sleep movement was the need for better obstetrics. De Lee, an ardent foe of twilight sleep, concluded in 1916 that the harm done by its use was "much overbalanced by the good accomplished." He referred to the:

> elevation of the standard of teaching and practice of obstetrics which has resulted from drawing public attention to the child-bearing woman, her sufferings, her needs. Without question we are having better obstetrics, and more of it than before 1914, and the seed will grow and the tree will spread.[132]

Indeed, the parallel reform movement initiated by obstetricians using twilight sleep as a vehicle had begun to bear fruit by the 1920s. Midwives were slowly regulated out of existence, and obstetricians, rather than general practitioners, moved in to fill the gap.[133] The twilight sleep movement gave critical impetus to obstetric reform.

The introduction of the twilight sleep into American obstetrics thus sparked a controversy, initiated a progressive reform movement, and served to encourage yet another reform movement. That the twilight sleep movement "failed" on its own terms was due to extensive professional opposition and limitations inherent in the technique itself. But the twilight sleep controversy served as a crucible for the formulation and realization of contemporary ideas about childbirth and obstetrics that were basic to the position of twilight sleep advocates.

Notes

1. Gen. 3:16.

2. John Duffy, "Anglo-American Reaction to Obstetrical Anesthesia," *Bulletin of the History of Medicine* 38 (1964): 32-44; Barbara M. Duncum, *The Development of Inhalation Anesthesia with Special Reference to the Years 1846-1900* (London: 1947); Claude E. Heaton, "The History of an Anesthesia and Analgesia in Obstetrics," *Journal of the History of Medicine* 1 (1946): 567-72.

3. Francis E. Kobrin, "American Midwife Controversy: A Crisis of Professionalization," *Bulletin of the History of Medicine* 40 (1966): 350-63.

4. Case records of the Boston Lying-In Hospital and the New England Hospital for Women and Children, Archives, Countway Library of Medicine, Boston, Mass. See Charles M. Steer, "Obstetrics at Sloane Hospital, 1891 and 1952," *Obstetrics and Gyneocologic Surgery* 9 (1954): 631-44.

5. See Kobrin, *American Midwife Controversy*.

6. W. B. Dewees, "Painless Labor, or the Status of the Means to Prevent Birth-pain," *International Medical Magazine* 3 (1894-1895): 794-812. See also, I. A. Shirley, "The Inhumanity of Refusing the Parturient Woman the Boon of Anesthesia," *Amer. Pract. and News* 36 (1903): 246-48.

7. Charles Jewett, ed., *The Practice of Obstetrics* (Philadelphia, 1901); J. H. Dye, *Painless Childbirth, or Healthy Mothers and Healthy Children,* 17th ed. (Buffalo, 1912); Albert Westland, *The Wife and Mother: A Medical Guide* (Philadelphia, 1892); William T. Lusks, *The Science and Art of Midwifery* (New York, 1899).

8. Andrew M. Claye, *The Evolution of Obstetric Analgesia* (London, 1939).

9. C. J. Gauss, "Geburten in Kunstlichen Dammerschlaf," *Archiv fur Gynakologie* 78 (1906): 579.

10. See Claye, n. 10, above; also Marguerite Tracy and Mary Boyd, *Painless Childbirth* (New York, 1915), pp. 99-100.

11. Tracy and Boyd, *Painless Childbirth,* p. 91.

12. F. S. Newell, "Anesthesia in the First Stage of Labor," *Surgery Gynecology and Obstetrics* 3 (1906): 126-30.

13. F. S. Newell, "Further Experiences with Scopolamine-Morphine Anesthesia in Obstetrics," *Surgery Gynecology and Obstetrics* (1907): 153-55.

14. W. H. Birchmore, "The Hyoscin Sleep in Obstetric Practice," *Medical Record* 71 (1907): 60.

15. Alfred M. Hellman, *Amnesia and Analgesia in Parturition* (New York, 1915), p. 104; Joseph B. De Lee, ed., *Obstetrics,* vol. 7 in the Practical Medicine Series, ed. Charles L. Mix (Chicago, 1907), p. 104.

16. De Lee, *Obstetrics,* p. 95.

17. Barton C. Hirst, *A Text-book of Obstetrics,* 7th ed. (Philadelphia, 1912), pp. 187-88.

18. Henry D. Fry, *Maternity* (New York, 1907), p. 138.

19. Bernhard Kronig, "The Difference Between the Older and the Newer Treatments by X-ray and Radium in Gynecological Disease," *Surgery Gynecology and Obstetrics* 18 (1914): 530.

20. Tracy and Boyd, *Painless Childbirth,* pp. 185-204.

21. M. Tracy and C. Leupp, "Painless Childbirth," *McClure's* 43 (1914): 37-51.

22. M. Boyd and M. Tracy, "More about Painless Childbirth," *McClure's* 43 (1914): 56-69.

23. Cited in E. M. Lazard, "The Twilight Sleep Propaganda in the Lay Press," *Southern California Practice* 30 (1915): 14.

24. Cited in A. L. Mann, "Is Twilight Sleep to Be 'for Me'. A Blessing—or a Curse?", *Illinois Medical Journal* 27 (1915): 265. Other articles include C. Leupp and B. J. Hendrick, "Twilight Sleep in America," *McClure's* 44 (1915): 25-37.

25. "Another 'Twilight Sleep'," *Literary Digest* 50 (1915): 187.

26. Cited in Ibid., p. 187; see also E. G. Zinke and J. O. Polak, "Has the Dammerschlaf a Place in General Practice," *Medical Times* 42 (1914): 343.

27. A. J. Rongy, "The Uses of Scopolamine in Labor," *American Medicine* 10 (1915): 45-49.

28. E. G. Zinke, in Zinke and Polak, "Has the Dammerschlaf a Place," p. 361; W. Gillespie, "Analgesics and Anesthetics in Labor, Their Indications and Contra-Indications," *Ohio Medical Journal* 11 (1915): 611.

29. "The Twilight Sleep," *Modern Hospital* 3 (1914): 255.

30. Kronig publicly denied complicity in twilight sleep publicity, which he described as inaccurate. The *McClure's* authors corroborated his statement. See "A letter from Dr. Kronig," *Literary Digest* 49 (1914): 507; Mann, "Is Twilight Sleep to Be 'for Me'," p. 265; A. C. King, "The Various Anesthetics as Applied to Obstetrical Work," *New Orleans Medical Surgical Journal* 64 (1911-1912): 662.

31. Hellman, *Amnesia and Analgesia in Parturition,* p. 7. Also W. H. Knipe, "The Freiburg Method of Dammerschlaf or Twilight Sleep," *Transactions New York Obstetrical Society* (1913-1916): 202; F. A. Dorman et al., "Special discussion with reference to twilight sleep by the request of the Committee on Public Health, Hospitals, and Budget of the Academy for a formal expression on this subject," *American Journal of Obstetrics* 71 (1915): 343.

32. Tracy and Boyd, *Painless Childbirth,* p. 120.

33. Ibid., p. xxxiii. See also R. K. Carter, *The Sleeping Car Twilight, or Motherhood without Pain* (Boston, 1915); Janna Rion, *The Truth About Twilight Sleep* (New York, 1915).

34. J. A. Harrar and R. McPherson, "Scopolamine-narcophin Seminarcosis in Labor," *Transactions American Association of Obstetrics and Gynecology* 27 (1914): 372-89.

35. Rion, *The Truth About Twilight Sleep,* p. 62. Tracy and Boyd, *Painless Childbirth,* p. 33.

36. Carter, *The Sleeping Car Twilight,* p. 36.

37. "'Authority' Spoke Too Soon!" *New York Times,* 24 August

1914, p. 8; "Accusing The Medical Profession," *New York Times,* 17 September 1914, p. 8; "An Answer Hardly Adequate," *New York Times,* 22 September 1914, p. 10; "Twilight Sleep Once More," *New York Times,* 7 November 1914, p. 10; "They Do So Hate Coercion," *New York Times,* 30 November 1914, p. 8.

38. " 'Twilight Sleep' Vindicated," *New York Times,* 20 October 1914, p. 12.

39. Carter, *The Sleeping Car Twilight,* p. 106. See also the papers of Dr. Eliza Taylor Ransom, Schlesinger Library, Radcliffe College, Cambridge, Mass.

40. William L. O'Neill, *Everyone was Brave: The Rise and Fall of Feminism in America* (Chicago, 1975), p. 187; Eleanor Flexner, *Century of Struggle: The Woman's Rights Movement in the United States* (Cambridge, Mass., 1959).

41. Benjamin V. Hubbard, *Socialism, Feminism, and Suffragism: The Terrible Triplets* (Chicago, 1915), p. 187; Margaret Stephens, *Woman and Marriage* (New York, 1910), p. xii.

42. Ellen Key, *The Woman Movement* (New York, 1912), p. 191.

43. Tracy and Boyd, *Painless Childbirth* p. 45. D. P. Reidy, "The Proper Management of Labor by the Physician," *Proceedings Connecticut Medical Society,* 123 (1915): 183-94. "Twilight Sleep," *Nation* 101 (1915): 211-12.

44. Tracy and Boyd, *Painless Childbirth,* p. 146; Rion, *The Truth About Twilight Sleep,* p. 30.

45. King, "The Various Anesthetics," p. 658; Gillespie, "Analgesics and Anesthetics in Labor,"; M. W. Kapp, "Painless and Shockless Childbirth, Twilight Sleep," *Medical Record* 90 (1916): 241.

46. F. S. Newell, "The Conduct of a Case of Labor," no date, in F. S. Newell, *Collected Papers,* Countway Library of Medicine, Boston, Mass.

47. G. E. Markowitz and D. K. Rosner, "Doctors in Crisis: A Study of the Use of Medical Education Reform to Establish Modern Professional Elitism in Medicine," *American Quarterly* 25 (1973): 83-107.

48. James Harvey Young, *The Medical Messiahs: A Social History of Health Quackery in Twentieth Century America* (Princeton, 1967).

49. Newell, "The Conduct of a Case of Labor," p. 2; Hellman, *Amnesia and Analgesia in Parturition,* p. 128.

50. Benjamin Rush, "On the Means of Lessening the Pains and Dangers of Childbearing," *The Medical Repository* (New York, 1803), 6: 26-7.

51. "Twilight Sleep," *American Medicine* 10 (1915): 1.

52. M. W. McDuffie, "Painless Childbirth from Observations of 'Twilight Sleep' or 'Dammerschlaf'," *North American Journal of Homeopathy* 29 (1914): 667.

53. Tracy and Boyd, *Painless Childbirth,* p. 64.

54. Henry Smith Williams, *Twilight Sleep* (New York, 1914), p. 10; Alice Hamilton, "Dammerschlaf," *Survey* 33 (1914): 158.

55. Dye, *Painless Childbirth,* p. 51.

56. Williams, *Twilight Sleep,* pp. 38-41.

57. George J. Engelmann, *Labor Among Primitive Peoples* (St. Louis, 1882), p. 7.

58. Dye, *Painless Childbirth,* p. 52.

59. Williams, *Twilight Sleep,* p. 39.

60. Dye, *Painless Childbirth,* pp. 18, 58, 60; Williams, *Twilight Sleep,* p. 90; Tracy and Boyd, *Painless Childbirth,* p. 25; S. F. B. Wakefield, "Scopolamin Amnesia in Labor," *American Journal of Obstetrics and Gynecology* 71 (1915): 428.

61. George W. Crile, *The Origins and Nature of the Emotions* (Philadelphia, 1915); John B. Huber, "The Newer Anesthesia," *Harpers Weekly* 58 (1914): 14; Williams, *Twilight Sleep,* p. 41.

62. Tracy and Boyd, *Painless Childbirth,* p. 29; C. H. Davis, *Painless Childbirth, Eutocia, and Nitrous Oxid-Oxygen Analgesia* (Chicago, 1916), p. 19; Kapp, *Painless and Shockless Childbirth,* p. 241.

63. Birchmore, "The Hyosin Sleep," pp. 59-60; Bertha van Hoosen, "The New Movement in Obstetrics," *Woman's Medical Journal* 25 (1915): 121.

64. See notes 10, 33, and 54 for more detailed presentations.

65. Harrar and McPherson, "Scopolamine-narcophin," p. 629; F. W. Lynch, "Eutocia by Means of Nitrous Oxid Gas Analgesia: A Safe Substitute for the Freiburg Method," *Journal of the American Medical Association* 64 (1915): 1187-89.

66. Lynch, Ibid., discussion.

67. Williams, *Twilight Sleep,* p. 18; Knipe, in Zinke and Polak, "Has the Dammerschlaf a Place," p. 362; Bertha van Hoosen, *Scopolamine-Morphine Anesthesia* (Chicago, 1915), pp. 99-100; Williams, *Twilight Sleep,* p. 25.

68. Hellman, *Amnesia and Analgesia in Parturition,* p. 161; R. M. Beach, "Twilight Sleep," *American Medicine* 10 (1915): 43.

69. W. H. W. Knipe, "Twilight Sleep from the Hospital Viewpoint," *Modern Hospital* 3 (1914): 250-251; Hellman, *Amnesia and Analgesia in Parturition,* pp. 76-77; Beach, "Twilight Sleep," p. 43.

70. Havelock Ellis, *The Task of Social Hygiene* (Boston, 1914); J. Halpenny and C. H. Vrooman, "The Use of Morphine and Scopolamine in Labor, with a Report of 200 Cases," *American Journal of Obstetrics and Gynecology* 60 (1909):612; George J. Engelmann, "The Increasing Sterility of American Women," *Journal of the American Medical Association* 37 (1901): 896.

71. Beach, in Knipe, "The Freiburg Method," p. 204; Knipe, in Zinke and Polak, "Has the Dammerschlaf a Place," p. 363.

72. Rion, *The Truth About Twilight Sleep,* pp. 14-18.

73. Tracy and Boyd, *Painless Childbirth,* p. 117.

74. Rion, *The Truth About Twilight Sleep,* p. 362.

75. W. H. W. Knipe, "Twilight Sleep: Its Future and Relation to General Practice," *American Medicine* 10 (1915): 32; Polak, in Zinke and Polak, note 36 above, 362.

76. Knipe, in Zinke and Polak, "Has the Dammerschlaf a Place," p. 362; J. O. Polak, "A Study of Twilight Sleep, with a Critical Analysis of the Cases at Long Island College Hospital," *New York Medical Journal* 10 (1915): 289; Davis, *Painless Childbirth,* pp. 55-57.

77. W. D. Beacham, "History of the Section on Obstetrics and Gyne-

cology of the AMA," *Journal of the American Medical Association* 169 (1959): 147-83; William F. Mengert, *History of the American College of Obstetricians and Gynecologists 1950-1970* (1971).

78. See Korbin, "American Midwife Controversy."

79. Davis, "Painless Childbirth," Preface, p. 57; Williams, *Twilight Sleep.*

80. J. W. Williams, "Medical Educations and the Midwife Problem in the U. S.," *Journal of the American Medical Association* 58 (1912): 1-7; J. W. Williams, "Why is the Art of Obstetrics So Poorly Practiced?" *Long Island Medical Journal* 11 (1917): 169-78; Williams, *Twilight Sleep,* pp. 73-82.

81. Tracy and Boyd, *Painless Childbirth,* p. 178; Van Hoosen, *Scopolamine-Morphine Anesthesia,* p. 283.

82. Leupp and Hendrick, "Twilight Sleep," p. 170; Tracy and Boyd, *Painless Childbirth,* pp. 43, 118.

83. Carter, *The Sleeping Car Twilight,* p. 176.

84. "Mothers Discuss Twilight Sleep," *New York Times,* 18 November 1914, p. 8.

85. "Twilight Sleep Triumphant," *New York Times,* 25 February 1915, p. 8.

86. Ransom papers, twilight sleep clippings scrapbook.

87. Leupp and Hendrick, "Twilight Sleep," p. 34; see also C. B. Ingraham, "Twilight Sleep," *Colorado Medicine* 12 (1915):13; New England Hospital for Women and Children, "53rd Annual Report, for 1915" (Boston, 1916), p. 17.

88. "West Holds Lead in Twilight Sleep," *New York Times,* 10 May 1915, p. 24.

89. Hellman, *Amnesia and Analgesia in Parturition,* pp. 119-23.

90. Tracy and Boyd, *Painless Childbirth,* p. 144.

91. Davis, *Painless Childbirth,* p. 59.

92. Rheta C. Dorr, *What Eight Million Women Want* (Boston, 1910); William L. O'Neill, ed., *The Woman Movement* (London, 1969).

93. *Buffalo Times,* 16 October 1914, cited in Ransom papers, twilight sleep clippings scrapbook.

94. Sources dealing with the National Twilight Sleep Association are Carter, *The Sleeping Car Twilight,* and the Ransom papers.

95. Carter, p. 181; Ransom papers, twilight sleep clippings scrapbook.

96. Ransom papers, twilight sleep clippings scrapbook.

97. Knipe's address attempted to refute arguments against twilight sleep (Ransom papers, twilight sleep file).

98. "Clinic for Twilight Sleep," *New York Times,* 8 February 1915, p. 4. See also "Twilight Sleep in Movies," *New York Times,* 26 August 1915, p. 9, for a description of a movie to promote twilight sleep. The NTSA had chapters in New England and the Midwest as well. Dr. Eliza Ransom was especially active. Ransom's career is well documented in scrapbooks and files preserved in the Ransom papers.

99. Ransom papers, twilight sleep file.

100. Case records, Boston Lying-In Hospital.

101. Ransom papers, twilight sleep clippings scrapbook.

102. Ibid., May 1915.

103. Ransom papers, twilight sleep file.

104. E. T. Ransom, "Twilight Sleep," Massachusetts *Clubwoman* 1 (1917): 5.

105. W. F. B. Wakefield, "Painless Childbirth," *American Journal of Obstetrics and Gynecology* 77 (1918): 796. See also van Hoosen, "The New Movement in Obstetrics," p. 122.

106. Samuel P. Hays, *Conservation and the Gospel of Efficiency* (Cambridge, Mass., 1959); Gabriel Kolko, *The Triumph of Conservatism* (New York, 1963); Robert H. Wiebe, *Businessmen and Reform, a Study of the Progressive Movement* (Cambridge, Mass., 1962); Robert H. Wiebe. *The Search for Order, 1877-1920* (New York, 1967).

107. *American Medicine* 10 (1915): 149.

108. "Safeguarding against Scopolamine Casualties," *Journal of the American Medical Association* 64 (1915): 598.

109. From the Ransom papers, twilight sleep file: "Drops Twilight Sleep," *New York Times,* 29 May 1915, p. 20; "Twilight Sleep Condemned," *New York Times,* 26 March 1915, p. 12.

110. Ransom papers, twilight sleep clippings scrapbook.

111. W. Livingston, "Scopolamine-morphine Amnesia in Labor," *American Journal of Obstetrics and Gynecology* 78 (1918): 549.

112. "Mothers Exhibit "Twilight" Babies," *New York Times,* 30 April 1915, p. 8.

113. Ransom papers, twilight sleep file.

114. "Doctors Disagree on Twilight Sleep," *New York Times,* 31 August 1915, p. 5.

115. "To Fight Twilight Sleep," *New York Times,* 25 August 1915, p. 10.

116. "Proclaiming a Poor Triumph," *New York Times,* 25 August 1915, p. 10.

117. See "Doctors Disagree on Twilight Sleep;" for statements of relief over its demise. See also De Lee, *Obstetrics,* p. 100; and J. Clifton Edgar, *The Practice of Obstetrics,* 5th ed. (Philadelphia, 1916), p. 838.

118. L. A. Le Doux, "Scopolamine-apomorphine Amnesia in Obstetrics," *Texas State Journal of Medicine* 21 (1925-1926): 422.

119. Bertha van Hoosen, "Scopolamine Anesthesia in obstetrics," *Current Research in Anesthesia* 7 (1928): 152.

120. H. Aranow, "A Post-mortem on Twilight Sleep," *New York Medical Journal* 108 (1918): 64.

121. Ibid., p. 65.

122. Livingston, "Scopolamine-morphine Amnesia in Labor," p. 553.

123. A. Brant, "Anesthesia in Obstetrics," *Boston Medical and Surgical Journal* 174 (1916); 458.

124. R. L. Raiford, "Painless Labor," *Virginia Medical Monthly* 50 (1923-1924): 152.

125. A. H. Bill, "The Choice of Methods for Making Labor Easy," *American Journal of Obstetrics and Gynecology* 3 (1922): 65.

126. H. W. Kostmayer, "A Practical Method of Minimizing the Pain of Labor," *New Orleans Medical and Surgical Journal* 69 (1916): 89.

127. W. C. Danforth and C. H. Davis, "Obstetric Analgesia and Anesthesia," *Journal of the American Medical Association* 81 (1923): 1090.

128. Aranow, "A Post-mortem on Twilight Sleep," p. 66.

129. Wakefield, "Painless Childbirth," p. 791.

130. H. Schwarz, "Painless Childbirth and the Safe Conduct of Labor," *American Journal of Obstetrics and Gynecology* 79 (1919): 46-63.

131. R. L. De Normandie, "Conservative Versus Radical Obstetrics," *Boston Medical Surgical Journal* 188 (1923): 1,028.

132. De Lee, *Obstetrics*, p. 100.

133. Kobrin, "American Midwife Controversy."

MARTHA H. VERBRUGGE

3　*The Social Meaning of Personal Health: The Ladies' Physiological Institute of Boston and Vicinity in the 1850s*

One of the more striking phenomena in American culture today is the growing interest in personal health. Perhaps more consciously than ever before in the twentieth century, Americans are seeking ways of achieving a higher degree of physical and emotional well-being. They do not lack resources. The popular media carry numerous descriptions of systems of diet, exercise, relaxation, and self-help medicine. Supplementary products, from special foods to exercise devices, are widely available. A person can seek fitness by joining a health spa or gym, learn about holistic living at private seminars and institutes, and find alternative medical care at self-help and sectarian clinics. Health has become as much a national preoccupation and profitable business as it is a deep personal concern.

While this growth of interest is indisputable, its origins are not as obvious. One wonders why concern for health is flourishing at this time and why it is most intense among Americans.On further reflection, one cannot help but speculate that some connection exists between the movement for personal well-being and the general temper of the period. The timing and political undertones of the health crusade have much in common with other movements of the 1960s and 1970s. For example, there has been rising dissatisfaction with the monopolistic structure of American medicine and the lack of quality health care.[1] More generally, opposition to our capitalist and technocratic system also has intensified in recent years. People

45

have sought alternatives that are economically more equitable and personally more fulfilling. Physical and psychic well-being figure prominently in their schemes. Finally, one of the first concerns raised by the present-day women's movement has been the right to control one's own body. The problems of abortion, rape and health care remain key issues among feminists.[2] Many recent political causes, then, have either built on or provoked a closer look at the way Americans view and handle the physical dimension of their lives.

Still, it is difficult to pinpoint the social and political meaning of Americans' interest in personal health. The puzzle becomes more manageable if one examines similar phenomena as they developed in the past. The current trend is not unique in either the annals of Western societies in general or American history in particular. One illustration is the interest in personal health that spread through the American Northeast during the middle decades of the nineteenth century. Although still considerably different from our own times, the history of that period is instructive. It may illuminate the origins and meaning of concern for personal health in American society.

Throughout the northeastern region of the United States the years between 1820 and 1860 were ones of enormous change.[3] The economic base shifted from a mixture of agriculture and commerce to a rudimentary but expanding system of industrial production. The population became increasingly urban and heterogeneous, as foreign immigrants joined native farmers and townspeople in crowded cities.

The structure of people's work and home life changed accordingly. Many activities and products of the home were transferred to factories. Hired to work at a factory or on piecework at home, ordinary people no longer controlled the means of production; they received a wage or its equivalent as compensation for their labor.[4] The industrial revolution also fostered the growth of a more prominent middle class. The production and distribution of goods required many secondary services. Urban areas attracted middle-rank proprietors, white-collar workers, and a variety of independent skilled tradesmen. Their prospects were rather tenuous. Although the bourgeoisie had a modicum of social stature and comfort, economic success and even minimum security were not certain.[5]

The same tension was evident in the family life of the urban middle class. On the one hand, women and children gained new opportunities. For example, bourgeois ladies were expected to enjoy the "freedoms" of shopping, social visiting, cultural outings, and even charitable and civic activities. At the same time the demands of supervising a good household increased. Once a self-sustaining unit, the family became the key agency in preparing individuals for their callings in life and for moderating the psychological and physical changes wrought by the outside world. In the process, women assumed a complex of both old and new responsibilities. More than ever before, the duties of the bourgeois wife and mother dealt with the management of home life and the socialization of future workers and citizens. In effect, the middle-class woman was both social gadabout and domestic cornerstone, both free and bound.[6]

The transformation of life during the mid-1800s did not happen smoothly. There was widespread concern about the personal and social implications of change; organized discontent grew and reform groups multiplied.[7] As wage-workers formed unions and various political groups, the middle and upper classes marshalled their forces as well. Some reforms, like abolition, seemed to focus on distant problems. Others were designed to intervene in the affairs of local, often lower-class, citizens. Elites supported public education, temperance, moral reform, and other causes in an effort to keep industrial and urban change under control.[8]

For some Americans, the answer to social disorder lay in the principles of Nature and the laws of health. Both human disease and social turmoil, they argued, originated in violations of natural law. The remedy, they concluded, was for people to learn and follow the paths of true living as revealed by the teachings of physiology and hygiene. This was the central message of what historians have called the popular health reform movement of the mid-nineteenth century. Advocates of the movement maintained that human health, if not perfection, was possible and that its attainment was contingent on the personal commitment of every American. Popular education in health and the awakening of personal conscience were the hallmarks of the health reform movement.[9]

Middle-class supporters enlisted every available means to spread their cause. The literature of the mid-1800s was filled with exhortations about health and with practical tips for daily life. Books, journals, and newspaper items about health proliferated. Special institutions for learning and practicing the ways of good health sprang up everywhere. They ranged from therapeutic centers, like water-cure spas in the countryside, to urban gymnasia that offered private instruction in exercise. Private and public schools introduced coursework in physiology, hygiene, and calisthenics. Public lectures and voluntary associations were organized to popularize "the laws of life and health."

Instruction in health was considered especially critical for women. After all, it was argued, women faced unique physiological problems throughout their lives; they also had to supervise the physical condition of their families and their homes. Moreover, health reformers continued, the hygienic and moral influence of women was likely to permeate society as a whole. Women were regarded as the models and the arbiters of sound living for those who worked or were preparing to serve in the world beyond the home. Thus, women's involvement was viewed as a vital component of personal health reform during the mid-1800s.[10]

The basic features of the cause were embodied in an organization founded in Boston in 1848, the Ladies' Physiological Institute of Boston and Vicinity.[11] The main work of this exclusively female association was the instruction of its members in the lessons of anatomy, physiology, hygiene, and other matters related to health and disease. As its constitution stated, "The objects of this Society are, to promote among *Women,* a knowledge of the HUMAN SYSTEM, the LAWS OF LIFE AND HEALTH, and the means of relieving sickness and suffering."[12]

The name of the Ladies' Physiological Institute was an apt one. First of all, "physiological" instruction was construed to mean the basics of human life, health, and disease. Through weekly lectures, a library, and a collection of models and charts, the Institute covered every lesson that "the science of human life" offered.[13] Members studied the rudiments of anatomy and physiology under such topics as the brain, respiration, and digestion. They learned about the source and care of specific diseases, including consumption, cholera, and typhoid fever. They were introduced to the principles of different medical and scientific systems, such as phrenology, hydropathy, and mesmerism.

Institute members anticipated that such knowledge would help them understand and thereby improve the human condition. Along with other health reformers, they regarded illness as an avoidable experience that persisted because of people's ignorance or neglect of natural law. They considered personal knowledge about the human system and its proper care as the first step toward health. As the secretary proclaimed to Institute members in 1857,

> You stand as a Physiological School, . . . the study of the human body, —to learn its structure, its functions, its derangements, —to learn the means to correct those derangements and to prevent suffering, —to learn the laws which govern life and health, are the pursuits to which your attention has been turned. What pursuits more ennobling? . . . As we look about us, on either hand, we see disease marking its prey; taking for its victim the budding infant, the blooming youth, as well as the man of declining years; and, as the funeral note strikes our ear, we catch the words, "Mysterious Providence!" and then all is silence. In view of such facts, it becomes us, who have been engaged in the study of the laws of life, —who have learned the sources from which disease must unavoidably issue, —who have traced effects to their cause, to awaken our energies, and once more renew our exertions to spread light upon subjects like these.[14]

Thus, according to the Institute, the principles of physiology were mankind's surest guide to personal health and happiness. In fact, members believed that physiological instruction also held significance well beyond physical life. Along with other health reformers, they declared that piety, moral rectitude, and social order would be served as well. Through the science of human life, they reasoned, people would witness God's "beautiful workmanship of [their] bodies" and acknowledge that a set of divine and immutable laws governed mankind's physical, mental, and spiritual natures.[15]

Moreover, the Institute regarded physiology as a means of opening "many avenues of reform."[16] The prevalence of sickness and premature death signaled for them a basic discord between human life and the divine plan. Physical degeneration was seen as both a cause and a symptom of disorder through-out modern life. Members hailed physiological knowledge as the panacea for moral and social decay as well as for personal ill-health. In 1852 the Institute's secretary forecast what kind of legacy the organization might leave:

> Although no structure of Granite or of marble shall be reared, to commemorate these our efforts, or mark the place of our first beginning, yet, a more noble structure shall be reared, shall appear in the ages, the structure of the human form, shall come forth, in its loveliness not as now, marked and marred by deformity, disease and suffering; but shall appear in its completeness, harmonious in its proportions, perfect in its developments, fitted and trained for usefullness. . . . The "Golden Age" is before us, and as a signal, we would present . . . our "Ladies' Physiological Institute" as destined to prepare the way, to usher in that golden period so long foretold by bard and sage; and in the fulness of time, bringing man into harmony with nature and with God.[17]

The key that Institute members held was their understanding of the condition and potential of mankind as revealed by physio-logical law.

The Institute's program reflected that broad conception of physiology. Along with talks on anatomy and pathology, mem-bers heard lectures on "Health & Religion," "Self Conquest," "Beauty," and "The Principles of Life." If the themes of the latter talk "were fully understood & brought to bear upon prac-tical life," the secretary noted after the meeting, "many of the existing evils of social life would be removed—and man brought into harmony with nature & with God again, resuming his pris-tine state, innocence and purity."[18] While such an observation sounds romantic today, it reflected the optimism and perfec-tionist vision that typified middle-class reform movements in America during pre-Civil War times.[19] The Institute believed that the level of popular physiology would raise individuals and society as a whole from a state of decay to one of health, order, and progress.

If the term "physiological" signified the women's concerns, their identity as an "institute" was equally fitting. During the ante-bellum period and later, the group's primary activity was its weekly meeting, conducted nine to twelve months of the year, despite bad weather and holidays. The Institute's reach did not extend much beyond its own membership. At times lectures were opened to the female public for a small admission fee, and, less often, free lectures were sponsored.[20] The Institute had no regular publication.[21] It conducted no fairs or literature campaigns devoted to popularizing physiology.[22] Except for its relations with outside speakers, the Institute rarely had close contact with other individuals or organizations.[23] During its early history the Institute was dedicated to group study and existed in virtual seclusion. That characteristic makes it stand out among other voluntary associations of the mid-nineteenth century. Many other middle-class reform groups used educational and interventionist means to effect change among their peers and among the lower class. The outward focus and public visibility of such campaigns were not shared by the Institute. Members were intent on quiet, personal study, With self-improvement as its animus, the Institute maintained a low profile for much of its early history.

The Institute's name offers one further clue about the group's design. "Ladies," sounded more refined than did "Women's" or "Female." The Institute prided itself on having a membership of "ladies of high intellectual culture, refined taste and moral excellence."[24] After just one year, 454 such women from the Boston area had joined. Although the total dipped to 130 by May 1854, it climbed to 300 by May 1857.[25] The Institute had 100 members in 1866 and, apparently, 500 in 1871.[26]

While the membership was large and respectable, it also was incredibly fluid. Although provisions for renewing membership were simple, between 23 percent and 57 percent of the women dropped out annually during the Institute's early years.[27] In 1857, the secretary reported that 1,015 different women had been members since the group's founding. "Of the three hundred members of to-day," she wrote, "not more than fifty have been with us more than three years."[28] Except for a core of durable members and officers, the Institute was composed mainly of respectable ladies whose participation was short-lived. The Institute's resiliency is a puzzle to the historian. On the one hand, the group was very dedicated, conducting its studies with remarkable scope and persistence. On the other hand, the Institute was seemingly fragile, a self-contained organization with a fluid membership. How did the Institute survive? What was the continuing appeal of a women's organization devoted to physiological instruction?

Though crucial, such questions are not readily answered. First, few details about Institute members are available. While some of the women were notable historical figures, the majority came from the more obscure population of nineteenth-century Boston. Few left personal records that would allow a historian to reconstruct the general patterns, let alone private details, of their lives. More generally, there is presently no historical model that satisfactorily explains phenomena such as the Institute. Our understanding of the organizations and experiences of middle-class urban women in ante-bellum times is still inadequate.[29]

Despite these limitations, one can develop a sense of the Institute's appeal. Besides the internal records that have survived, there are a number of sources and techniques to help fill in a sketch of the organization. In recent years social historians have developed a number of tools that uncover many details about relatively anonymous urban populations. Source materials include census reports, church records, city directories, and other municipal data. Initially, historians focused on patterns of nativity, occupation, and mobility among urban men, whose activities seemed more visible and thereby amenable to study.[30] Many of the same resources and techniques can be used, with some difficulty or modification to study the lives of urban women.[31] The following profile of the Ladies' Physiological Institute is based primarily on information from city directories, supplemented by municipal lists of major taxpayers, a mapping of residences, and obituaries of members or their husbands in local newspapers.[32]

The starting point was a published list of members for the Institute's first year, 1848 to 1849.[33] A trace of the women revealed that the early membership consisted primarily of white, non-working, married or widowed women whose husbands were middle class to upper-middle class. Of the 385 women listed, approximately 60 percent came from Boston proper or the nearby harbor towns of South Boston and East Boston.[34] Seventy-five percent were either married or widowed, as indicated by their designation as "Mrs." on the list; perhaps only 5 percent were actually widows. Some 7 percent of the members held jobs; most of those who did work were in acceptable "female" areas such as teaching, medicine, and dressmaking.[35] The other women were the wives or daughters of men in the middle class or upper-middle class.[36] Among the Boston cohort, for example, nearly 80 percent of the members' husbands or fathers were either merchants or skilled artisans of fairly comfortable means.[37] Another 15 percent of the men were professionals or white-collar workers.

Occupation alone does not measure a person's economic or social standing. Another index is the value of one's personal and real property, which is reflected in annual tax assessments. During the ante-bellum period the city of Boston published lists of persons and corporations who paid taxes above a certain level. Comparing those lists with the Institute's membership, one can conclude that a modest number of the Boston members came from wealthy families. A significant percentage (10 to 20 percent) appeared on the tax lists during the 1840s and 1850s, but few claimed property holdings that qualified them as upper class.[38] Their economic prospects were tenuous, however; it was never certain whether one's standing would rise or fall from year to year.[39]

A final measure of the members' situations is residence. The women tended to live in districts that were predominantly middle class during the mid-1800s.[40] Those areas included the south and west "ends" of the city proper, as well as East Boston and South Boston. Only a few resided in such fashionable areas as Beacon Hill or in the increasingly immigrant working-class districts like the North End.

If the general membership represented the substantial middle class, the leadership of the Institute was simply a smaller sample. A reading of the group's records from the 1850s produced a list of the Institute's most active and durable members.[41] Seventy-five percent were married or widowed. Over three-quarters live in the city proper, East Boston, or South Boston.[42] This residential cohort came from comfortable and even well-to-do families engaged in business or skilled trades.[43] It also included fifteen women who worked and five widows, or 11 percent and 4 percent, respectively, of the Boston subgroup.[44] Certain women did tend to concentrate in the Institute's various leadership positions. At the core was a group of married women from middle- to upper-middle-class families who served as the primary officers (president, vice-president, and secretary).[45] At their side was the board of directors, a group of fifteen women who helped oversee Institute affairs. In many cases the most regular board members were women whose husbands or fathers were well-to-do. A number of widows, wives, and daughters from Boston's elite served for four to six of the Institute's first nine years.[46] They were joined by a group of long-term board members who came from less prosperous but still substantial families. Finally, a number of special members rose quickly through the Institute's ranks. They included local medical practitioners, such as Harriot Kezia Hunt and Martha A. Sawin,[47] and well-known authors and reformers, such as Caroline H. Dall and Carolina M. Severance.[48]

The general membership and leaders of the Institute were a special slice out of Boston's population at mid-century. The group was weighted heavily toward the middle ranks of the city's economic and social hierarchy. It is therefore likely that the women shared certain expectations and experiences. At the same time, the Institute was not a homogeneous group. There were significant differences in terms of marital status, duration of membership, and degree of contacts and visibility in the city at large. The question remains as to what drew this particular collection of women together. What personal and social functions did the Institute serve for its varied membership?

A possible answer emerges as one looks at the dynamics of the Institute more closely. The women were not a random sample from Boston's middle class. A significant number were the relatives, neighbors, or friends of other members. In fact, the organization included some complicated networks of female friends.[49] Moreover, the loss of key members, when they moved away or died, was felt deeply. In 1851, for example, the secretary reported that, "as a band of sisters," the Institute had sent its sympathy to the families of two deceased members. Such condolences, she noted, demonstrated "that the association of scientific interests extended to the more endearing & intimate relation of affectionate & sympathizing regard for each other's joys & afflictions."[50] A warmth pervaded the organization, which may have sustained its older members and attracted new ones. That feeling of sorority was probably an extension of the companionship that Institute women enjoyed in other settings. From the diary of a leading member, it is evident that Institute members frequently exchanged visits, shopped together, and attended cultural events with each other.[51] As neighbors and kin, they probably shared intimate experiences in their homes as well.

The vitality of female association was not new in the mid-nineteenth century. Nor was it confined to voluntary organizations like the Institute. Sorority in many forms had been an integral part of women's lives in America for a long time.[52] Nevertheless, it took on new dimensions in the mid-1800s in the context of urban and industrial life. Though domestic duties still prevailed, the bourgeois life opened new roles and opportunities for women. Various outings and organized activities in the company of other women became increasingly acceptable. The economic and social structure of Boston allowed, if not depended upon, the more sociable pastimes of women.[53] The Institute legitimized that arrangement. It helped build a network in which members shared problems, expectations, and friendship; it also provided evidence of and reinforcement for the patterns of respectable middle-class life.

Boston offered numerous formal settings in which women could associate. Nevertheless, many women chose to join the Institute, however briefly. There is no doubt that membership was deliberate. A cross-check between the Institute and a variety of other organizations in ante-bellum Boston revealed few overlaps. For many women, in other words, the Institute was a rare if not unique social activity.[54]

The special appeal of the Institute is not hard to ascertain. Physiological information was immediately useful for the middle-class urban woman. It laid out practical guidelines for personal care, domestic management, and the other responsibilities that filled a woman's daily agenda. The nurture of family members and the maintenance of a healthy home environment had become major obligations, if not a woman's true "profession." As the fabric of domestic life changed in ante-bellum times, women were assigned ever more responsibility and authority as the managers of the home. Problems related to health and disease were central to the expectations and realities of "true womanhood." The Institute helped its members accommodate. Called by Nature and society to oversee health, women were now equipped by science to handle their duties effectively.

The exchange of reliable information, in an open and caring atmosphere such as the Institute's, must have been a welcome opportunity.[55]

The Institute was designed to serve the members' daily needs. Though diverse, its program addressed the major problems that the women faced in their homes and personal lives. The library housed many guides to help wives and mothers with their daily responsibilities. Talks on the management of infants and the sick were quite popular. On 30 October 1850, for example, Harriot K. Hunt lectured on "The Temperaments." According to the minutes, Hunt "alluded to the wrong management of mothers & others having charge of youth, & pointed out the responsibility resting on those who have been enlightened on the subject of Physiology, to counteract the tendencies of present customs."[56] The Institute also studied questions of a more personal nature. A number of talks in the 1850s offered advice about personal hygiene and daily habits. The topic of women's dress was especially lively.[57] Other lectures, as well as library books, covered the subjects of childbirth and female physiology. For example, Orson Squire Fowler, the noted phrenologist, talked about midwifery and parturition.[58] Dr. Ezra W. Gleason, a homeopath delivered a lecture on "the cessation of the Menses, or the turn of life."[59]

It does not appear, however, that the Institute encouraged frank discussion of such matters as birth control and marital relations. In 1850, for example, Dr. Frederick Hollick, a rather infamous proponent of sex education, donated some of his books to the Institute's library. Regarding the subject matter too sensitive and even dangerous for uninitiated minds, the Institute placed "the books in the hands of the [Board of] Directors, to be lent by them to such persons as their judgement approved."[60] The Institute chose to address its members' needs as mothers and women with a discretion befitting their class and times.

Members appreciated the practical value of the Institute's work. Useful information, it appears, was the main expectation and benefit of membership. Institute members accepted prevailing norms of womanhood without question. They agreed that, by design and circumstance, women were responsible for the well-being of their families and, by extension, of society and the race. "The mother has been termed a sculptor, in view of her influence on mind and character," observed the Institute secretary in 1850.[61] Members viewed physiology as the body of theoretical and practical knowledge that would best equip them to mold the lives of their charges. The Institute, remarked the secretary in 1850, "is eminently adapted to our wants, & is designed to provide the kind of instruction, which will fit us for an intelligent performance of our duties, as wives, mothers, nurses, & guardians of youth."[62]

In fact, the members saw their power as extending beyond the domestic circle to society at large. As the secretary explained in 1851:

> The information imparted at our lectures, the results of scientific research, & laborious study, presents a large amount of highly valuable knowledge, of practical utility, pre-eminently useful to the mother, in the care of her family, & affecting the welfare of a large part of the community, —for who can estimate the influences exerted by Woman, through the minute radiii [sic] of the *home circle*—instruction to her in the necessity of reform is felt worldwide, if her heart responds to the teachings.[63]

Institute members shared with other reformers the conviction that physical and moral improvement was the special province of women.

Whether their attention settled on daily chores or the broader goal of human progress, Institute women found physiological instruction a useful guide. The Institute helped its members cope with the demands of daily life. In a period of rapid change and uncertainty, the Institute outlined the roles of the middle-class-urban woman and gave her instruction in how to meet her responsibilities. In social terms, the Institute helped legitimize the expectations and realities of women's lives. In personal terms, each member may have returned home with a body of authoritative knowledge and greater self-confidence.

Although its impact was generally conservative, the Institute did have radical potential. Outside speakers may have exposed members to new and political ideas. Lecturers included such women as Lydia F. Fowler and Paulina W. Davis, who popularized physiology throughout New England in the mid-1800s; they were also prominent in such movements as women's rights, abolition, and temperance.[64] Some of the Institute's more distinguished members also represented ways of life and thought

57

that were uncommon among middle-class women.[65] Finally, one of the group's few outside contacts in the 1850s involved the drive for women's medical education. Around mid-century a number of efforts began in the Northeast to train women in medicine. Though its support was modest and tentative, the Institute did express interest in the medical programs for women in Boston and New York.[66]

Through associations such as these, Institute members faced challenges to the usual pattern of middle-class and female life. Though few embraced what they saw and heard, some members were changed by the experience. For a minority, the Institute probably extended or even provoked new insights about women's lives and American society. In some cases the Institute was a stepping stone to other public activities. Mrs. Eunice H. Cobb, a founder and long-time member, for example, expanded on her appearances before church groups and the Institute and became a popular speaker on religious and physiological topics around New England during the 1860s and 1870s.[67] In some ways, then, the Institute was a daring experiment. Though generally unfulfilled, the potential for a feminist or radical course did exist.

The Institute is not on trial, however. If the members "failed" to endorse radical change, they did so for reasons that were persuasive within the context of their lives and times. For the urban middle class, conditions at mid-century presented an uneasy reality. Though comfortable, the economic and social position of Institute families was precarious. Wedged between the lower class and the elites, the middle class accepted the new economic structure while they preserved a culture of familiar values and norms. Domestic order and stability represented an antidote to the less manageable forces of the outside world. Personal health reform, in particular, assumed great significance as a means of self-control and self-improvement. Although many strategies for social and political reform were open during ante-bellum times, an accessible and direct solution may have been especially attractive to bourgeois Bostonians. The supervision of personal habits and domestic hygiene was a modest investment that promised enormous dividends.[68]

The Institute contributed to that process. It helped legitimize women's roles and reinforced the ideology that self-management, perseverance, and domestic cohesiveness were the founda-

58

tions of success in an otherwise uncertain world. The philosophy and work of the Institute channeled the concerns of members and their families into the quiet area of self-reform. Education and personal conscience, not social reorganization, were accepted as the best agents of stability and progress. The Institute both directed and served the needs of its middle-class female members and their families in ante-bellum Boston.

The Ladies' Physiological Institute still exists, making it the oldest continuous women's organization in America today. It has changed considerably over the last one hundred years. No longer the vanguard of physiological instruction and health reform, it is a small, well-established group of older women. Its primary business is quarterly sociables and the donation of funds to various scholarships and charities.

It is not inconceivable that the Institute will return to its original design, for, in some ways, present-day conditions resemble those in which the Institute was founded. It began in a period of social and political upheaval; the themes of holistic living and personal responsibility were widely espoused; the conviction that women had special needs and obligations in the area of health was common.

Such factors did not guarantee that the Institute would follow a progressive course. The conservative development of the group may deliver a message to those who are interested in personal health reform today. Although it has enormous value and even radical potential, present-day concern for personal care and fitness is not free from dangerous implications. Already commercial interests are exploiting the movement for private profit. Moreover, the ideology of personal responsibility is both welcome and oppressive. While motivating self-control, it labels all behavior as individual triumph or failure, to the exclusion of political or economic factors. Finally, current notions about what constitutes health and how one achieves it reinforce cultural norms and social divisions. According to class, sex, race, and age, each person is expected to seek a particular state of health through a prescribed regimen of life. As the history of the Institute suggests, the social origins and meaning of personal health are neither arbitrary nor timeless. Nor are the constraints within today's movement inevitable if we recognize and act upon the broad political dimensions of "health."

Notes

1. Recent critiques include Barbara and John Ehrenreich, *The American Health Empire: Power, Profits, and Politics* (New York: Random House, Vintage Books, 1971); and David Kotelchuck, ed., *Prognosis Negative: Crisis in the Health Care System* (New York: Random House, Vintage Books, 1977).

2. For example, see Boston Women's Health Book Collective, *Our Bodies, Our Selves* (New York: Simon and Schuster, 1973; rev. ed., 1976); and Claudia Dreifus, ed., *Seizing Our Bodies: The Politics of Women's Health* (New York: Random House, Vintage Books, 1978).

3. General background sources include Arthur M. Schlesinger, Jr., *The Age of Jackson* (Boston: Little, Brown & Co., 1945); George R. Taylor, *The Transportation Revolution, 1851-1860* (New York: Rinehart and Company, 1951); and Edward Pessen, *Jacksonian America: Society, Personality, and Politics* (Homewood, Ill.: The Dorsey Press, 1969).

4. The changing nature of work is considered in Caroline F. Ware, *The Early New England Cotton Manufacture: A Study in Industrial Beginnings* (Boston: Little, Brown & Co., 1931; reprint ed., New York: Russell and Russell, 1966); and Herbert G. Gutman, "Work, Culture and Society in Industrializing America, 1815-1919," *American Historical Review* 78 (1973): 531-88.

5. For interesting studies in this field, see Stephan Thernstrom and Richard Sennett, eds., *Nineteenth-Century Cities: Essays in the New Urban History,* Yale Studies of the City, (New Haven: University Press, 1969).

6. The character of bourgeois womanhood and family life is discussed in Barbara Welter, "The Cult of True Womanhood, 1820-1860," *American Quarterly* 18 (1966): 151-74; Gerda Lerner, "The Lady and the Mill-Girl: Changes in the Status of Women in the Age of Jackson," *Mid-Continent America Studies Journal* 10 (1969): 5-15; Ann G. Gordon, Mari Jo Buhle, and Nancy Schrom, "Women in American Society: An Historical Contribution," *Radical America* 5 (1971): 3-66; Mary P. Ryan, *Womanhood in America: From Colonial Times to the Present* (New York: New Viewpoints, 1975); and Nancy F. Cott, *The Bonds of Womanhood: Woman's Sphere in New England, 1780-1835* (New Haven: Yale University Press, 1977).

7. A general survey is found in Alice Felt Tyler, *Freedom's Ferment* (Minneapolis: University of Minnesota Press, 1944; reprint ed., New York: Harper & Row, Harper Torchbooks, 1962). Interpretive essays include John L. Thomas, "Romantic Reform in America, 1815-1865," *American Quarterly* 17 (1965): 656-81; and Gerald N. Grob, "Modernization and Traditionalism in Social Reform," in *Men, Women & Issues in American History,* eds., Howard H. Quint and Milton Cantor, 2 vols. (Homewood, Ill.: Dorsey Press, 1975), 1: 192-214.

8. For example, see Clifford Griffin, "Religious Benevolence as Social Control, 1815-1860," *Mississippi Valley Historical Review* 44 (1957): 423-44; and Michael B. Katz, *The Irony of Early School Reform: Educational Innovation in Mid-Nineteenth-Century Massachusetts* (Cambridge,

Mass.: Harvard University Press, 1968).

9. Secondary literature about the "popular health reform movement" of the mid-1800s include surveys like William B. Walker, "The Health Reform Movement in the United States, 1830-1870" (Ph.D. diss., Johns Hopkins University, 1955); and John B. Blake, "Health Reform," in *The Rise of Adventism: Religion and Society in Mid-Nineteenth-Century America,* ed. Edwin S. Gaustad (New York: Harper and Row, 1974), pp. 30-49. A broader interpretation, under the new label of "personal health reform," may be found in Verbrugge, "Fitness for Life: Female Health and Education in Nineteenth-Century Boston" (Ph.D. diss., Harvard University, 1978).

10. The most recent studies of this theme include Verbrugge, "Fitness for Life," and two pieces by Regina Markell Morantz: "Nineteenth-Century Health Reform and Women: A Program of Self-Help," in *Medicine Without Doctors: Home Health Care in American History,* eds., Guenter B. Risse, Ronald L. Numbers, and Judith Walzer Leavitt (New York: Science History Publications, 1977), pp. 73-93; and "Making Women Modern: Middle Class Women and Health Reform in 19th Century America," *Journal of Social History* 10 (Summer 1977): 490-507.

11. This study focuses on the first decade of the Institute's history. (A more complete account of that and later periods may be found in Verbrugge, "Fitness for Life." This article is based primarily on the surviving records of the Ladies' Physiological Institute, housed at the Arthur M. and Elizabeth Schlesinger Library on the History of Women in America, Radcliffe College, Cambridge, Massachusetts. Hereafter that collection will be cited as LPI and individual manuscript volumes will be designated as I (Minutes, January 1850-January 1851); II (Minutes, January 1851-May 1854); III (Minutes, May 1854-May 1857); IV (Board Minutes, January 1851-April 1857); and V (Treasurer's Book). Yearly reports in the records are denoted simply as "2nd Ann. Rept.," "3rd Ann. Rept.," and so on. Other sources for this study include published reports, official documents of the group, and various local materials, such as city directories, tax assessment listings, and obituaries in newspapers.

12. Article I of the Constitution, printed in *Synopsis of the Proceedings of the Second Annual Meeting of the Ladies' Physiological Institute, of Boston and Vicinity, with the Secretary's Report, and the Constitution and By-Laws of the Society, with Catalogue of Library* (Boston: Alfred Mudge, Printer, 1851), p. 13 (hereafter cited as *Sec. Ann. Meeting*).

13. Meetings consisted of invited speakers or group discussions, called "conversationals." The library, which housed 330 volumes by May 1857, included medical and popular health journals, books on physiology, hygiene, and disease, and works on natural history and social philosophy. The Institute listed its scientific apparatus and models in *Sec. Ann. Meeting,* p. 12.

14. *Ninth Annual Meeting of the Ladies' Physiological Institute, May Sixth, 1857* (Boston: Alfred Mudge & Son, 1857), p. 11 (hereafter cited as *Ninth Ann. Meeting*).

15. "2nd Ann. Rept., LPI, I: 51; *Sec. Ann. Meeting,* p. 9.

16. "3rd Ann. Rept.," LPI, II: 46-47.

17. "4th Ann. Rept.," LPI, II: 137-37 (the volume has two pages numbered "137"); pp. 134-138 in general.

18. LPI, III: 21 January 1857.

19. See n. 7, above, especially Thomas, "Romantic Reform.'"

20. During the 1850s the price ranged between ten and fifteen cents per person. Paid attendance averaged between ten and twenty people and sometimes ran as high as fifty. Free lectures were introduced in 1850-1851, when six were given.

21. Despite early promises, the Institute printed only a few of its annual reports. The possibility of editing a popular journal or tracts about physiology and health was never raised.

22. During its first ten years the Institute did hold a number of fund-raisers to improve the group's finances. According to some members, however, such events did little to uphold the Institute's principles or stature.

23. The group heard from representatives of every popular system of medicine and science, including regular physicians, hydropaths, homeopaths, botanics, mesmerists, and phrenologists. The relationships that developed (and some were intimate and long-term) were based on mutual interests rather than the institutional or professional connections of the speaker.

24. *Ninth Ann. Meeting,* p. 9.

25. Membership figures were noted in the secretary's annual reports. From May 1849 to May 1857, the yearly percentages of growth or decline were: -34 percent, +7 percent, -26 percent, -27 percent, -24 percent, +18 percent, +14 percent, and +70 percent.

26. Both of these figures appear in the diary of Mrs. Eunice Hale Cobb (1803-1880), a founder, president, and long-time guiding spirit of the Institute. (Her personal memoirs are located in the Rare Book Department of the Boston Public Library, Boston, Massachusetts.)

27. Women retained membership by paying annual dues (fifty cents in the early years and one dollar by 1857). Turnover rates were calculated from information in the annual reports concerning total membership and new membership. After five years the number of dropouts stabilized between 12 and 18 percent.

28. *Ninth Ann. Meeting,* p. 9.

29. However, historical work in this field is growing constantly. General studies include Eleanor Flexner, *Century of Struggle: The Woman's Rights Movement in the United States* (Cambridge, Mass.: Harvard University Press, Belknap Press, 1959; rev. ed., 1975); Keith E. Melder, *The Beginnings of Sisterhood: The American Woman's Rights Movement, 1800-1850* (New York: Schocken Books, 1977); and Barbara Berg, *The Remembered Gate: Origins of American Feminism - The Woman and the City, 1800-1860,* Urban Life in America series (New York: Oxford University Press, 1978). Detailed investigations of particular women or groups have also been done in such areas as moral reform and religious charities.

30. The male population of Boston, for example, has been examined in the pioneering work of Peter R. Knights in *The Plain People of Boston, 1830-1860: A Study in City Growth* (New York: Oxford University Press, 1971); and Stephan Thernstrom in *The Other Bostonians: Poverty and*

Progress in the American Metropolis, 1880-1970, Harvard Studies in Urban History (Cambridge, Mass.: Harvard University Press, 1973).

31. Exemplary contributions include two papers presented at the Third Berkshire Conference on the History of Women, Bryn Mawr College, Bryn Mawr, Pennsylvania, 9-11 June 1976: Marlou Belyea, "New England Female Moral Reform Society, 1837-1850"; and Susan Porter Benson, "Women, Networks and Reform: Providence Employment Society, 1837-58" (now published in *Journal of Social History* 12 (Winter 1978): 302-13.)

32. Nineteenth-century directories gave considerable information about the work and domestic situations of a city's adults. Yet they were selective and often unreliable. Directories are both useful and limited in historical studies about urban women. Since most bourgeois women were neither workers nor heads of households, the position of many Institute members had to be inferred by locating information about their fathers or husbands. For more details about this method, see Verbrugge, "Fitness for Life."

33. See *Ladies' Physiological Institute—Semi-Centennial Report. In Memoriam—Salome Merritt, M.D.* (n.p., n.d.), pp. 9-19 (hereafter cited as *Semi-Cent. Rept.*). This list gives the names of 385 members from the first season and, in most cases, their street and/or town addresses.

34. The rest came in clusters of fifteen to thirty women from nearby communities (such as Cambridge and Charlestown) and in smaller groups of two to five women from such places as Brighton and Somerville.

35. These figures are minimums since they were calculated on the basis of total membership, whether located or not. Ninety percent of the workers were single, representing 17 percent of all single women in the organization.

36. The class label signifies both a qualitative and quantitative judgement. The men were first categorized according to the occupational scheme used by Knights in *The Plain People,* pp. 149-56. A second measure was level of wealth, using the scales suggested in the city's annual records of tax assessments and Knights' work on Boston.

37. Thus, the Institute was not a microcosm of Boston. According to Knights' sample of heads of households from the 1850 census, less than half of the city's residents came from those general occupational groups (calculated from Table V-1, p. 84, of *The Plain People*).

38. The 230 Boston residents were matched against the city's tax lists of 1842 (City Document No. 9), 1847 (No. 12), and 1855 (No. 22). Some members were relatively wealthy, as judged by the cutoff of $10,000 in property value that Knights used to separate upper-middle-class from upper-class taxpayers.

39. Of the families who appeared on both the 1842 and 1847 lists, 90 percent had increased tax assessments. For the comparable group between 1847 and 1855, 86 percent enjoyed greater holdings. At the same time, success (by this measure) was increasingly slippery. While 91 percent of those on the 1842 list reappeared in 1847, only 74 percent from 1847 were listed in 1855.

40. See Knights, *The Plain People,* pp. 13-18; Walter Muir Whitehill, *Boston: A Topographical History* (Cambridge, Mass.: Harvard University

Press, 1959; 2d ed., 1968); and Sam Bass Warner, Jr., *Streetcar Suburbs: The Process of Growth in Boston, 1870-1900* (Cambridge, Mass.: Harvard University Press, 1962).

41. The manuscript records revealed the names of 750 women, and 256 of those were pulled out. Selections were based on level of participation and amount of personal information (full name and address). Therefore, the sample was skewed toward the most active or distinctive members, including officers, committee members, and doctor-members.

42. This figure is based on the number of women in the sample for whom addresses were found, that is, 175.

43. Sixty-four women in the Boston subgroup were traced through a male family member. A majority of the men were modest or wealthy proprietors (44 percent) or tradesmen (22 percent). The rest were white-collar workers (11 percent) or professionals (9 percent).

44. Twenty-seven women in the Boston subgroup had independent directory listings because they headed a household or worked. The workers held jobs in such "respectable" areas as teaching, medicine, dressmaking, and art.

45. The first president was a man, Charles P. Bronson, an elocutionist and lecturer who helped found the Institute. He was succeeded by Mrs. Eunice Hale Cobb (n. 26, above), the wife of a leading Universalist minister and editor, who served as president in 1850, 1853-1855, and 1860-1862. The vice-president was usually the wife or widow of a local merchant. The two secretarial posts were often held by unmarried women. Three women served as treasurer between 1848 and 1857, including the wife of a clergyman and the wife of a prosperous globe maker.

46. The married women included the wives of a dry goods proprietor, a shipbuilder, a provisions dealer, and a die-sinker. A striking number of widows and single women from wealthy families also served from one to seven years on the board.

47. Harriot K. Hunt (1805-1857) was president in 1856 and 1857. She was a self-taught medical practitioner and a social activist who supported popular instruction in physiology, women's suffrage, and the anti-slavery movement. (See her autobiography, *Glances & Glimpses* [Boston: John P. Jewett, 1856], and a biographical sketch in *Notable American Women,* 2: 235-37). Mrs. Sawin (1815-1859), a charter member, was president in 1858 and 1859. She was among the first graduates of the Boston Female Medical College. See Frederick C. Waite, "Dr. Martha A. (Hayden) Sawin: The First Woman Graduate in Medicine in Practice in Boston," *New England Journal of Medicine 205* (26 November 1931): 1053-55.

48. Mrs. Dall (1822-1912) was a noted author and women's rights leader in the Boston area throughout the second half of the nineteenth century (see *Notable American Women,* 1: 428-29). Mrs. Severance (1820-1914) led a similarly active life as a reformer and lecturer, especially on behalf of women's rights and abolition (see *Notable American Women,* 3: 265-68).

49. The published list of original members, the admissions records of the 1850s, and a residential mapping clearly demonstrate that many members were connected in some way. They joined in such combinations as

mother-daughter(s), sister-sister, and next-door neighbors. Often women with identical surnames and/or similar addresses were proposed for membership at the same meeting, joined shortly thereafter, and then extended the network by drawing even more friends into the Institute. Recently other scholars have found similar networks in various female organizations of the mid-1800s; for example, see the references in n. 31, above.

50. "3rd Ann. Rept.," LPI, II: 38.

51. Cobb's diary, vols. 2-5, BPL (n. 26, above).

52. See Carroll Smith-Rosenberg, "The Female World of Love and Ritual: Relations Between Women in 19th-Century America," *Signs* 1 (Autumn 1975): 1-29.

53. See the references in n. 6, above.

54. A number of groups whose memberships were primarily or exclusively female were checked. Examples include the Boston Female Anti-Slavery Society, the Boston Children's Friend Society, and the City Missionary Society. (However, Institute women may have joined other groups well before or after the 1850s.)

55. The domestic roles of bourgeois women are discussed in the works cited in n. 6, above, and in Kathryn Sklar, *Catharine Beecher: A Study in American Domesticity* (New Haven: Yale University Press, 1973). The work of Morantz (n. 10, above) develops a similar argument about health reform and middle-class women. Morantz focuses on the psychological and practical value of scientific knowledge at a time when roles were vague and preparation was inadequate.

56. LPI, I: 109.

57. Reports of lectures and discussions about dress are found in LPI, I: 95, II: 41, 220.

58. LPI, II: 89, 98.

59. LPI, II: The recording secretary made special note of "the delicacy with which he treated the subject."

60. LPI, I: 71-72 (12 June 1850), I: 74 (2 July 1850).

61. "2nd Ann. Rept.," LPI, I: 52; *Sec. Ann. Meeting*, p. 9.

62. "2nd Ann. Rept.," LPI, I: 51-54; *Sec. Ann. Meeting*, pp. 9-10.

63. "3rd Ann. Rept.," LPI, II: 47.

64. Lydia Folger Fowler (1822-1879) held a degree from the Central Medical College in Syracuse and was married to Lorenzo Niles Fowler, a popular phrenologist (see *Notable American Women*, 1: 654-55). Paulina Wright Davis (1813-1876) was another itinerant lecturer on health who supported abolition and women's suffrage (see *Notable American Women, 1; 444-45*). A number of lesser known women also addressed the Institute. They included an itinerant lecturer from the Midwest, a local mesmerist, the operator of an anatomical museum, and a local regular physician.

65. See notes 47 and 48 above.

66. While it denied having any formal connection, the Institute was close to several of the founders and faculty members of the Boston Female Medical College, established in 1848. At the urging of two pioneering female physicians, Dr. Marie Zakrzewska and Dr. Elizabeth Blackwell, the Institute donated some articles to a fundraiser for a medical school for women in New York City in 1856.

67. As the wife, and later widow, of a leading minister, Mrs. Cobb attended numerous meetings of the Universalist church and delivered many sermons and general talks. She also spoke before various groups on physiology and health. Her lectures carried her as far as Saratoga Springs, New York, Dover, New Hampshire, and Bridgeport, Connecticut. Mrs. Cobb's diaries record not only her busy schedule of talks but also her sense of anxiety and of personal growth as a speaker before large groups.

68. A similar argument has been made by William Coleman in "Health and Hygiene in the *Encyclopédie*: A Medical Doctrine for the Bourgeoisie," *Journal of the History of Medicine* 29 (October 1974): 399-421. Coleman argues that the very ideology and habits of personal hygiene were accessible to only a certain social stratum in revolutionary France. Thus, health was a means of both insuring and demonstrating the unique qualities of middle-class life.

VIRGINIA G. DRACHMAN

4 The Loomis Trial: Social Mores and Obstetrics in the Mid-Nineteenth Century

Throughout the nineteenth century changes in medical science, professional status, and medical education were central to the concerns of American physicians. The shift from lay midwifery to male-dominated obstetrics, the faltering professional status of doctors, and the need for reform in the organization, content, and method of medical education often engendered heated, acrimonious debates among practitioners. Sometimes these debates overflowed into the public arena, through newspaper articles or other means, and became intertwined with public attitudes toward health, disease, and even female modesty. The libel trial in 1850 of Dr. Horatio N. Loomis, a private practitioner in Buffalo, was one such event that attracted widespread public attention.[1] In this trial physicians were called upon to debate the value of a controversial pedagogical innovation—demonstrative midwifery, the practice of allowing medical students to observe women in labor as part of their training. But, through their testimony, doctors' concerns over much larger health-related issues surfaced quickly: the demise of midwifery and the establishment of obstetrics as a legitimate field of medicine for male physicians, the relationship of doctors to the larger community, and the relationship of private practice to medical education and hospital practice. "As connected with the introduction of a mode of teaching," noted the *Buffalo Medical Journal* at the time, and "as involving medical ethics, and affording indications of medical sentiment of the

I would like to thank Douglas Jones for his thoughtful criticism and advice.

present time, the trial will rank among the events which make up the history of medicine."[2] This chapter examines the trial within the general context of the history of nineteenth-century American medicine.[3]

The events leading up to the trial began in January 1850, when Dr. James Platt White, professor of obstetrics at Buffalo Medical College, allowed his students to observe while he attended a woman in labor. As the fetal head emerged from the pubic arch, approximately twenty students watched him remove some of the patient's clothing to demonstrate the proper technique for supporting the perineum. This was the first time in the United States that medical students had been permitted to observe a delivery. White's students were aware of the importance of this first incidence of demonstrative midwifery, and they publically praised their instructor in a written statement sent to the *Buffalo Medical Journal.*[4] Subsequently, one of the city's general newspapers, the *Buffalo Commercial Advertiser* published an editorial in support of demonstrative midwifery.[5] Shortly thereafter, an article critical of demonstrative midwifery appeared in another newspaper, the *Buffalo Courier.* The author, a Buffalo physician who identified himself merely as "L.," charged White with offending the modesty of the female patient by exposing her to the "meritricious curiosity" and "salacious stare" of his students and thereby committing a "gross outrage upon public decency" for the purpose of furthering his own professional reputation.[6] In response, Professor White's students issued another statement in his support.[7] To quiet the mounting controversy, the faculty of the college published their own statement of support, claiming that White's clinical instruction furthered "the interests of the students in their acquisition of useful knowledge, and, thereby, the interests of medical science and of humanity."[8] Meanwhile, Dr. Horatio Loomis, a private practioner suspected of being "L.," purchased additional copies of the critical letter that had appeared in the *Courier* and distributed them to citizens of Buffalo. To save his reputation, White brought Loomis to trial for libel, ultimately losing the case because he could not prove that Loomis was the author of the newspaper article.

Although White lost the case, this single incident of demonstrative midwifery signaled a major medical advance, for it set the stage for the routine practice of ocular deliveries in medical schools, a necessary precondition for the development of modern obstetrics. But there were many doctors who denounced demonstrative midwifery, defining it as medically unethical, pedagogically unnecessary, and professionally unsound.[9] In the mid-nineteenth century, after all, obstetrics as a legitimate area of medical practice for male physicians was not universally accepted among either lay people or doctors themselves. Until the mid-eighteenth century childbirth was understood to be a uniquely female experience that took place amidst female friends and relatives under the direction of the female midwife. Toward the end of the eighteenth century male physicians began to gain access to the delivery room. Some returning from Europe with new medical skills, and others having attended lectures in cities such as Boston and New York on the subject of midwifery, made themselves available as accoucheurs in complicated or dangerous cases. The presence of the skilled male accoucheur implied a changing attitude toward childbirth. No longer was it seen simply as an event of nature. Instead, it began to be understood as a complex physiological process that, often required the medical expertise of a trained physician. The implication that scientific knowledge and skill were now deemed necessary to avoid the dangers of childbirth set the stage for the eventual discrediting of midwives and for the legitimization of the skilled obstetrician.[10]

By the time of the Loomis trial it was not so unusual for male physicians, particularly in the urban centers of Boston, New York, and Philadelphia, to attend women in labor. Nevertheless, the male physician's position as accoucheur was far from secure. The midwife still presented formidable competition for him, for many women continued to prefer to deliver surrounded by female relatives, friends and the midwife. Male physicians seeking access to the delivery room were haunted by this tradition. "It is indeed, in our remembrance," explained one doctor, "that the very presence of a male practitioner in the house was scarce endured."[11] In addition to the persistence of the tradition of midwifery, women were beginning to break into the medical profession by 1850, competing with male physicians for access to the delivery room. Two women's medical colleges had already been founded, the New England Female Medical College and the Women's Medical College of Pennsylvania, and Elizabeth Blackwell had completed her instruction at Geneva Medical College and become the first woman to graduate from a regular medical school in the United States. The takeover of the delivery room by the male obstetrician was a process that took almost two centuries to complete.[12]

While by mid-century most male physicians seemed to agree on the validity of the male accoucheur, they disagreed over how he should behave in the delivery room. The male physician was expected to act simultaneously as both doctor and gentleman. As a doctor, his duty was to provide the best medical service possible to his patient. As a gentleman, however, he was expected to preserve the dignity and modesty of the woman. Dr. D. Humphreys Storer, professor of midwifery at Harvard, explained in his introductory lecture to the medical class of 1855-1856 that the female patient "does expect that uniformly gentlemanly deportment, that constant kindness, that fidelity, which ever characterize the true physician."[13] These dual responsibilities often placed the physician in a difficult dilemma of conflicting professional and social roles.

This problem was not new to male physicians. They had been facing it throughout the nineteenth century as they increasingly sought female patients. It manifested itself, for example, as doctors began to rely on the new instruments of medical technology in treating women. When some physicians began to use the vaginal speculum, for instance, many others resisted the innovation. By the time of the Loomis trial this controversy was in full swing. Routine use of the speculum was denounced by many because it involved an ocular examination of the female genitalia, a radical deviation from the traditional mode of examining female patients. Throughout the first half of the nineteenth century physicians had relied primarily on their sense of touch when they gave an internal examination; some looked at the female genitals in an emergency. Yet most generally agreed that to both look at and touch the female genitals unnecessarily, as in the case of a routine examination was to sacrifice female delicacy and ignore medical ethics. The influential Dr. Charles D. Meigs, professor of medicine and diseases of women and children at Jefferson Medical College in Philadelphia, was one doctor who urged restraint in the use of the speculum and reliance on it only when absolutely necessary. To Meigs, indiscriminate use of the speculum was an affront to female modesty and virtue. In fact, he explained that the doctor's primary obligation was not to fulfill his professional responsibility to heal the sick but to fulfill his social responsibility to preserve the moral fabric of society. Meigs explained this to his medical students:

> It is perhaps best, upon the whole, that this great degree of modesty should exist even to the extent of putting a bar to researches, without which no very clear and understandable notions can be obtained of the sexual disorders. I confess I am proud to say that in this country generally, certainly in many parts of it, there are women who prefer to suffer the extremity of danger and pain rather than wave those scruples of delicacy which prevent their maladies from being explored. I say it is fully an evidence of the dominion of a fine morality in our society.[14]

Demonstrative midwifery met similar resistance because, like the speculum, it involved exposing the female genitalia to the male eye. Previously medical students had learned about the birth process from pictures in books. Unless they had received some practical training as an apprentice, they usually would not have observed a delivery until they were practicing on their own. Most physicians and medical educators of the day considered this an adequate system of training. They believed that to allow students to observe a woman in labor for the purpose of instruction was unnecessary and therefore offensive to the modesty and virtue of the expectant mother. Loomis's attorney expressed these sentiments in his opening statement to the jury. "The exposure of this woman in labor," he charged, "was . . . a startling and bestial innovation. . . . Against the exposure of this woman," he continued, "we do protest. And we expect that you will by your verdict vindicate the delicacy of the sex."[15]

Even those doctors who championed demonstrative midwifery understood the importance of respecting the modesty of their female patients. White himself had heeded traditional medical etiquette and taken special precautions to protect his patient from the indiscriminate stares of his students. When the fetal head presented itself, he had covered the perineum with napkins while he demonstrated the proper method of supporting the perineum. From the testimony of the students it appears that their view of the patient's genitals had been effectively obscured. One student stated that "her genitals were not exposed."[16] Another testified:

> I didn't see any of the front part of her body. As the clothes were raised, I saw something in the form of flesh and blood; what it was I couldn't say. . . .I don't recall whether one or both hands supported the perineum. Professor White had a napkin in his hand. The woman was covered when the placenta was delivered.[17]

The students also testified that proper decorum had been preserved. In response to the charge in the letter by L. that the patient had been subjected to the "meretricious curiosity" and "salacious stare" of "a score of scarcely adolescent youth," one student explained that "the best of order was preserved in the room. I don't recollect any talking except between Professor White and the nurse."[18] Another student described the atmosphere in the room in more detail:

> There was no talk, unless the woman wanted something. There was no talk among the students.—There was no laughing or jesting. I saw one smile. Dr. White talked about the labor, for the purpose of instructing the class, his talk had no other tendency than to instruct the class. Professor White enjoined decorum and order. The house, as I said before, was still.[19]

White and his students clearly believed that demonstrative midwifery could take place without violation of female modesty and virtue.

Despite the differences of opinion expressed at the trial, there seems to have been an underlying consensus among the doctors there regarding the importance of preserving female delicacy and virtue. Yet the doctors also seemed to share the understanding that one could modify this principle of preserving female virtue. While they spoke about respecting the virtues of womanhood in general, it appears that they were most concerned about upholding the virtues of middle-class and upper-class women. They loosened their rigid standards when the woman in question was poor. White's patient, Mary Watson, for example, was a recent immigrant from Ireland, an unmarried woman living in the Erie County poorhouse. From the testimony of the physicians at the trial one sees hints of a double standard of medical practice whereby such women because of their ethnicity, economic condition, and marital status, were treated differently from more well-to-do female patients. One physician testified, for example, that he would "be fearful of introducing [demonstrative midwifery] into a private institution" and that in his "private practice he never expose[d] the female."[20] Another stated that "there ought to be a difference made between medical instructions to a class and private practice," that he "considered them entirely different," and that he "would not pretend to make the ladies in private practice the means of instruction to classes."[21]

We may better appreciate this way of thinking if we examine the response of physicians to demonstrative midwifery within the context of their relationship to the community. Because their access to the delivery room was far from absolute, doctors understood that what went on behind its door was by no means a purely private matter. They realized that the community at large was watching closely as they attended women in childbirth. Each uneventful, successful delivery they attended could heighten their reputations as respectable accoucheurs and further justify their presence in the delivery room. Similarly, any type of complication or event of note, such as demonstrative midwifery, could damage their reputation and destroy the uneasy alliance they were building with female patients. Hence, physicians resisted demonstrative midwifery in part because they feared that it would attract unfavorable attention and engender public controversy that would keep women away from them.

Throughout the trial doctors revealed their concern about the response of the community at large to the practice of demonstrative midwifery. They continually echoed the theme that demonstrative midwifery was "prejudicing the moral sense of the community against doctors."[22] One physician, a graduate of the University of Pennsylvania and a practicing physician for twenty-two years, explained:

> I disapprove of [demonstrative midwifery] . . . for the same general reason that has been stated here—it is contrary to the moral sense of the community. It is a principle in Medical Ethics, not to do anything to excite the public against the Medical Profession. Gregarious teaching in midwifery is improper.[23]

Another practicing physician of twenty-seven years echoed that "according to Medical Ethics, all unnecessary acts are to be avoided which are calculated to excite the public or create a prejudice against the profession."[24]

In seeking to maintain the favor of the community, physicians were particularly concerned about their relationship with female members of well-to-do families, who held the key to male physicians' entrance into obstetrics. Their allegiance and support could guarantee lucrative private obstetric practices and at the same time lend legitimacy and respectability to the major shift from midwifery to obstetrics.[25] For these reasons male doctors were careful not to offend well-to-do women as they sought to woo them into becoming their obstetric patients. Thus they adapted their medical behavior to conform to social etiquette.

Five years before the Loomis trial, this same fear of alienating the women of well-to-do families had prompted Boston physicians to reject a proposal to provide clinical instruction in midwifery for medical students at the Massachusetts General Hospital. The committee reviewing the proposal concluded that wealthy women, as well as self-respecting poor women, would refuse to tolerate such exposure. They argued that if the hospital lost the patronage of its respectable female patients, it would also lose the philanthropic support of the wealthy members of the Boston community. Like physicians in Boston, those at the Loomis trial feared demonstrative midwifery would destroy their delicate alliance with the community as they sought to strengthen their hold on the field of obstetrics.

The concern expressed by the physicians who testified at the Loomis trial should also be seen within the context of the public's general dissatisfaction with regular doctors. Physicians at mid-century were attempting to establish a strong professional identity and a comfortable relationship with the lay public. Their efforts were complicated, however, by the public's growing disenchantment with doctors' ineffective and often harmful therapeutics. By the end of the first third of the nineteenth century, this disenchantment had mushroomed into the rejection of regular medicine by large portions of the public, the growth of numerous medical sects offering alternatives to regular medicine, and a willingness among lay people to rely on these medical alternatives.[26] Though the challenge to regular medicine had

peaked before mid-century, public disrespect for it and enchantment with medical sectarianism were still riding the crest of
that peak at the time of the Loomis trial. Regular doctors, who
deemed themselves the only respectable medical representatives,
were in a quandary as to how to best cope with this assault. One
response was the establishment of the American Medical Association in 1848. Among its initial tasks, the AMA sought to
improve medical education, standardize medical practices,
and regulate the numbers of regular physicians. In so doing,
the American Medical Association sought to upgrade the public
image of regular physicians and to strengthen their defense
against medical sectarians. We may, therefore, understand the
uproar among doctors over demonstrative midwifery as growing
in part out of these attempts by regular physicians to monitor
and to regulate their own medical practices.

We may also appreciate it if we place it within the context of
regular doctors' attempts to distance themselves from the public at large. As part of their attempt to gain greater respect from
the community and improve their professional image, they
sought to distinguish themselves as different from lay people. In
so doing, they increasingly came to see medical issues as their
concern alone. Public input was deemed inappropriate. Thus,
for some of the doctors at the Loomis trial, the significant issue
was not so much White's demonstration of delivery to his students but the public discussion of it. "I do not think the trans-
action at the College as objectionable as the publication of it,"
explained one physician.[27] A colleague of White's explained
that, while he had assented to White's demonstrating a delivery
to his students, he had "not advise[d] the publication of the
Demonstration."[28] Similarly, another of White's colleagues
testified, "[I] don't so much object to its publication in a medical journal as in a secular newspaper, which I condemn *in
toto.* "[29] It was the article in the *Buffalo Commercial Advertiser*
in defense of demonstrative midwifery that he thought was "in-
judicious." The American Medical Association echoed these
sentiments in its report on demonstrative midwifery:

> It is to be regretted that this subject has been brought at all upon the
> popular arena. It is wholly a professional question, and should be
> discussed by the profession in a calm, considerate and dignified man-
> ner. It is no subject for newspaper warfare, nor for a warfare in
> medical journals in newspaper style.[30]

75

A single physician at the trial voiced a minority opinion. He explained that generally he would "disapprove of a publication in a secular newspaper, like that in the *Commercial*. But in this case it was different—the public mind had become excited on this subject, and that article was published for the purpose of allaying the excitement. . . ."[31]

The controversy over demonstrative midwifery was also a response to the changing standards of medical education. In the first half of the century most physicians were trained by apprenticing themselves to practicing doctors. Despite its popularity, this system of apprenticeship presented a variety of problems, There was, for example, no adequate way of regulating standards of medical education. Instead, the training of each individual medical student varied, depending on the knowledge and skill of his particular preceptor. In addition, as medical science progressed, the preceptor grew increasingly less competent to provide sufficient medical training.[32]

While most physicians in the first half of the nineteenth century had been trained by means of the apprenticeship system, some went to medical schools. The wealthier students either went to schools in Europe or to American medical schools such as the Philadelphia Medical College, Kings College in New York City, and Harvard, all of which had been founded during the last third of the eighteenth century and modeled after the schools in Europe. Other students attended any of the more local and less prestigious medical schools that had been growing in numbers throughout the nineteenth century. Not surprisingly, the quality of education varied greatly from school to school, and the lack of a standard program of medical education was one of the major problems of medical school training in the early nineteenth century. Another serious problem was that medical schools omitted what the apprenticeship stressed, practical training. The students' learning experience in medical school was confined almost solely to lectures; clinical and laboratory instruction were rare. Unless a student went to medical school and apprenticed himself to a physician as well, there was no way for him to get both theoretical knowledge and practical experience. The debate over demonstrative midwifery was part of the mid-century reevaluation among doctors of medical school education and particularly of the value of clinical training.

While this atmosphere of self-improvement had opened the door for reforms in medical education, we should not be surprised that physicians resisted introducing demonstrative midwifery into medical schools. Historically, resistance had been a predictable response to innovation among doctors. In the seventeenth century, for example, they had greeted the theory of circulation of the blood with much skepticism; in the eighteenth century they responded similarly to the practice of innoculation; and at the same time that Dr. White was trying to bring changes to the teaching of obstetrics, physicians were adamantly resisting new ideas regarding the contagious nature of puerpural infection.[33]

The resistance of physicians to demonstrative midwifery also was a defensive response in part for they realized that to acknowledge its pedagogical value was to concede the inadequacy of their own training experience. Thus physicians at the Loomis trial insisted that the traditional mode of learning obstetrics, by studying plates of the female anatomy and by tactile internal examination, was entirely sufficient. One physician, for example, explained that "the student can learn the distention of the perineum properly only by the sense of touch. The external parts can as well be seen upon plates as by ocular demonstration."[34] With plates, explained another physician, "the student can have all the parts before him at once, both of the internal and external organs; while he cannot have the living subject before him, except at long intervals. . . . The plates are almost perfect, exhibiting all the stages of labor during parturition."[35]

Those supporting the innovation of demonstrative midwifery responded quite differently. White's students were overwhelmingly in its favor, testifying that their instructor had given them a valuable learning experience that greatly enhanced their understanding of the birth process. "In my opinion," one explained, "demonstrative midwifery is important and useful as a means of imparting valuable instruction."[36] Another testified that he had "derived such confidence as to enable [him] to proceed better when called to attend a sick bed,"[37] while another explained that the ocular demonstration had "impressed upon his mind the *practical* part of what he only knew before by theory."[38]

White's graduates were not the only witnesses to speak in favor of the pedagogical benefits of demonstrative midwifery.

77

Practicing doctors also testified as to its value. Several of this latter group were men whose training had taken them to European cities such as Edinburgh, Paris, and Amsterdam, where demonstrative midwifery was an integral part of medical education. Their testimony in favor of the practice may have been particularly significant because many American doctors then believed European medicine was superior to American medicine and wished to use it as a model for American medical practice.[39]

The debate over demonstrative midwifery was not contained within the walls of the Erie County courtroom; doctors throughout the country participated in the controversy, carrying on the debate in their numerous medical journals, echoing the same themes of concern as those expressed by the doctors at the trial. Addressing the need for reform in medical education, for example, a letter from a physician to the *Boston Medical and Surgical Journal* praised White for "his endeavors to make the instruction in his department as practicable as possible."[40] Similarly, another doctor explained in the *New Orleans Medical Journal* that "our teachers of medicine have heretofore, devoted too much of their lectures to theoretical medicine to turn out competent graduates; practical *clinical* teaching will ultimately triumph. . . ."[41] In chiding the profession for resisting reform in medical education, one doctor surmised that the Buffalo physicians opposing demonstrative midwifery were members of the "opposition factions, so commonly found surrounding and impeding medical schools."[42] Another doctor, in a letter of support to the *New York Journal of Medicine,* reminded his colleagues that "novelty in practice . . . always meets with opposition" and asked, as an illustration that reminds us of the insecurity male doctors felt regarding their relationship to female patients, "who does not recollect the bitter persecution which attended the introduction of the stethescope (not to mention the speculum) into general practice, and the more than bitter persecution which was encountered by the early male-practitioners of obstetrics?"[43]

A letter to the *Charleston Medical Journal and Review* addressed this issue of reform of medical education as well as the issue of the autonomy of the medical profession from the public:

[I]f an attempt to do in this country, what has been quite common In Europe for years past, it is to be ground down by the mischievous uprising of the ignorant and uneducated, merely because it seems repugnant to their sense of what is fit—if the laity are to determine the *quid deciat* for the Medical Profession, then we had better content ourselves with lying down supinely, and waiting for their sanction, before attempting any improvements, however recommended by the progress of science, the advance of an enlightened civilization, or even the long experience of others.[44]

In a letter to the *Louisville Medical Journal* a doctor addressed both of these concerns as well as the question of the responsibility of physicians to uphold female virtue. He labeled the opposing physicians the "prudish Miss Nancies of Buffalo" and chided them for "their excessive modesty and shamefacedness."[45]

With demonstrative midwifery evoking such a nationwide controversy, it is interesting to look at the reaction of the newly formed American Medical Association. At its third annual meeting in 1850, the Association decided to undertake an investigation of "whether any practicable scheme can be devised to render instruction in Midwifery more practical than it has hitherto been in the medical schools of the United States."[46] Curiously, the Committee on Education was assigned the task of investigation rather than the Committee on Obstetrics, even though both committees agreed that the latter would have been the more appropriate investigating group. Unfortunately, the transactions of the meeting do not indicate the motives behind this decision. However, the very fact that this task fell to the Committee on Education suggests that the *AMA* preferred to define demonstrative midwifery primarily as an educational issue rather than as one of obstetric practice. In its report the following year, the Committee on Education rejected demonstrative midwifery first and foremost as an unnecessary and inadequate form of instruction. "We not only object to the mode of instruction, adopted in the plan at Buffalo, as unnecessary," the committee explained, "but we object to it, also, as being utterly *incompetent to give the student* that knowledge which he needs in the practice of obstetrics."[47] In addition, it was sensitive to the obstetric issues as well and expressed deep concern about the impact of demonstrative midwifery on the relationship between male doctors and female patients:

> The confidential relation existing between women and our profession, so essential to the full and proper treatment of her diseases, may be impaired either by the practices of individuals, or by those which may prevail very generally in the profession. Great carefulness, therefore, is needed on this point. The object, both of the individual practitioner and of the profession, should be to meet most fully the demands of science and humanity, and yet not offend a sensitive, but rational delicacy, nor give countenance to an unblushing shamelessness.
>
> It is principally the prejudice which indelicate practices among medical men have engendered in the public mind, that has given rise to the project for training female practitioners of medicine.[48]

In effect, the medical profession's major vehicle for promoting medical policy in the nation had rejected an innovation that many physicians throughout the country had greeted with great acclamation. The voice of caution in the face of change, the American Medical Association thus revealed the tenuous position of the medical profession as it sought to treat women. Its conservatism, however, was contrary to the winds of progress. The editor of the *New Orleans Medical Journal* correctly forecast the future when he wrote about demonstrative midwifery: "Practical clinical teaching will ultimately triumph over those who oppose it as alike grossly offensive to morality and common decency."[49]

In the post-Civil War period doctors evolved a working, though unspoken agreement with the growing population of poor urban women, not unlike Mary Watson. They gave them medical attention, and, in return, used them as a resource for medical instruction. Within a relatively short period of time after the Loomis trial, demonstrative midwifery became an acceptable mode of medical instruction among doctors as well as the public. Within this context, the Loomis trial gives us a snapshot of physicians during a period of transition as they struggled to come to grips with issues that would shape medicine for generations to come: establishing a female clientele, improving their professional relationship with the public, and reforming medical education.

Notes

1. Frederick T. Parsons, *Report of the Trial, The People versus Dr. Horatio N. Loomis, for Libel* (Buffalo: Jewett, Thomas and Co., 1800); also reprinted in Charles Rosenberg and Carroll Smith-Rosenberg, eds., *The Male-Midwife and the Female Doctor* (New York: Arno Press, 1974). An original publication of the report is in the archives at SUNY, Buffalo. The best copy of the report is the Arno Press reprinted edition, from which all quotes in this paper are taken.

2. *Buffalo Medical Journal and Monthly Review of Medical and Surgical Science* 6 (July 1850): 115.

3. Other historians have recognized the significance of the Loomis trial in the history of American obstetrics: Jane Donegan, "Midwifery in America, 1760-1860: A Study in Medicine and Morality" (Ph.D. diss., Syracuse University, 1972); Herbert Thoms, *Chapters in American Obstetrics* (Springfield: Charles C. Thomas, 1961); and Richard Wertz and Dorothy C. Wertz, *Lying-In: A History of Childbirth in America* (New York: The Free Press, 1977), pp. 85-89.

4. *Buffalo Medical Journal* 5 (February 1850): 565, reprinted in *Report of the Trial,* appendix, p. 42.

5. *Buffalo Commercial Advertiser,* 19 February 1850, reprinted in *Report of the Trial,* appendix, p. 43.

6. *Buffalo Courier,* 27 February 1850, reprinted in *Report of the Trial,* appendix, pp. 44-45.

7. Written statement by graduates of Buffalo Medical College session of 1849-1850, 15 February 1850, *Report of the Trial,* appendix, 43-44.

8. Resolutions of the Faculty of the Medical Department of the University of Buffalo, 26 February 1850, *Report of the Trial,* appendix, p. 44.

9. Seventeen Buffalo physicians publically denounced demonstrative midwifery in a letter to Dr. Austin Flint, Dean of the Buffalo Medical College and editor of the *Buffalo Medical Journal.* The letter appeared in *Buffalo Medical Journal* 5 (March 1850): 621 and in *Boston Medical and Surgical Journal* 42 (29 May 1850): 349, reprinted in *Report of the Trial,* appendix, p. 44.

10. For a discussion of midwifery in early America and the changing attitudes toward childbirth, see Catherine M. Scholten, " 'On the Importance of the Obstetrick Art': Changing Customs of Childbirth in America, 1760-1825," *William and Mary Quarterly* 34 (1977): 426-45.

11. *American Journal of the Medical Sciences* 20 (October 1850): 449.

12. For evidence of the resistance to the move toward obstetrics, see Samuel Gregory, *Letters to Ladies, in Favor of Female Physicians* (New York: Fowlers and Wells, 1850), reprinted in Rosenberg and Smith-Rosenberg, *The Male-Midwife and the Female Doctor* (New York: Arno Press, 1974); Samuel Gregory, *Man-Midwifery Exposed and Corrected: or, The Employment of Men to Attend Women in Childbirth, and in Other Delicate Circumstances Shown to be a Modern Innovation* (Boston: G. Gregory, 1848), reprinted in *The Male-Midwife and Female Doctor;* and

George Gregory, *Medical Morals: Illustrated with Plates and Extracts from Medical Works; Designed to Show the Pernicious Social and Moral Influence of the Present System of Medical Practice, and the Importance of Establishing Female Medical Colleges, and Educating and Employing Female Physicians for Their Own Sex* (Boston: 1853), reprinted in *The Male-Midwife and Female Doctor.*

13. David Humphreys Storer, *An Introductory Lecture Before the Medical Class of 1855/56 of Harvard University* (Boston: David Clapp, 1855), p. 11.

14. Charles D. Meigs, *Females and their Diseases* (Philadelphia: Lea and Blanchard, 1848), cited in James V. Ricci, *The Development of Gynaecological Surgery and Instruments* (Philadelphia: The Blakiston Co., 1949), p. 313.

15. *Report of the Trial*, p. 9.

16. Ibid., p. 9.

17. Ibid., p. 10.

18. Ibid., p. 10.

19. Ibid., p. 9.

20. Ibid., p. 27.

21. Ibid., p. 29.

22. Ibid., p. 14.

23. Ibid., p. 15.

24. Ibid., p. 16.

25. A physician, D. W. Cathell, expressed this understanding in a book on how to establish a successful medical practice that was widely read by doctors toward the end of the nineteenth century. D. W. Cathell, *The Physician Himself and What He Should Add to the Scientific Acquirements,* ed. Charles E. Rosenberg (New York: Arno Press, 1972).

26. For a discussion of the low esteem of the medical profession and the use of sectarian medicine, see, for example: William Rothstein, *American Physicians in the Nineteenth Century: From Sects to Science* (Baltimore: Johns Hopkins University Press, 1972); Richard Harrison Shryock, *Medicine and Society in America: 1660-1860* (Ithaca, N.Y.: Cornell University Press, 1960); Richard Harrison Shryock, "The American Physician in 1846 and in 1946: A Study in Professional Contrasts," *Medicine in America* (Baltimore: Johns Hopkins Press, 1966); and Richard Harrison Shryock, "Sylvester Graham and the Popular Health Movement, 1830-1870," *Medicine in America* (Baltimore: Johns Hopkins Press, 1966).

27. *Report of the Trial*, p. 15.

28. Ibid., p. 26.

29. Ibid., p. 27.

30. "Report of the Committee on Education in Relation to 'Demonstrative Midwifery' " submitted at the fourth annual meeting of the American Medical Association, in *Transactions of the American Medical Association* (Philadelphia: Collins, 1851) 4: 436-37.

31. *Report of the Trial*, p. 29.

32. On medical education, see, for example, William Rothstein, *American Physicians in the Nineteenth Century: From Sects to Science* (Baltimore: Johns Hopkins University Press, 1972); and Shryock, *Medicine and*

Society in America: 1660-1860.
33. *Report of the Trial,* p. 6.
34. Ibid., p. 13.
35. Ibid., pp. 12-13.
36. Ibid., p. 19.
37. Ibid., p. 20.
38. Ibid., p. 20.
39. See Shryock, *Medicine and Society in America: 1660-1860.*
40. *Boston Medical and Surgical Journal* 42 (29 May 1850): 258.
41. Editorial, *New Orleans Medical Journal* 6 (May 1850): 809.
42. *Cincinatti Medical Journal,* May 1850, reprinted in *Report of the Trial,* appendix, p. 48.
43. *New York Journal of Medicine and the Collateral Sciences,* 4 (May 1850): 395.
44. *Charleston Medical Journal and Review* 5 (September 1850): 672.
45. *Louisville Medical Journal,* June 1850, quoted in Thoms, *Our Obstetrical Heritage,* p. 108.
46. *Minutes of the Third Annual Meeting of the American Medical Association, Transactions of the American Medical Association* (Philadelphia: Collins, 1850), 3: 42.
47. "Report of the Committee on Medical Education in Relation to 'Demonstrative Midwifery,' " submitted at the fourth annual meeting of the American Medical Association, *Transactions of the American Medical Association* (Philadelphia: Collins, 1851), 4: 440.
48. Ibid., p. 440.
49. Editorial, *New Orleans Medical Journal* 6 (May 1850): 809.

JUDITH WALZER LEAVITT

5 *Politics and Public Health: Small Pox in Milwaukee, 1894-1895*

Smallpox was to Milwaukee what cholera and yellow fever were to other nineteenth-century American cities. It was an infrequent visitor, but when it came smallpox caused major disruptions of city life and generated fear and panic among the residents. The effects of smallpox epidemics were typically to increase the powers and effectiveness of the health department. John Duffy, Charles Rosenberg, and others have indicated this pattern with regard to cholera and yellow fever epidemics.[1] It also explains the impact of smallpox in Milwaukee. As a result of five nineteenth-century smallpox epidemics, health officials greatly increased their authority to control infectious diseases in Milwaukee.[2]

However, the smallpox epidemic that hit Milwaukee in the summer and fall of 1894 interrupted this pattern. As a direct result of that epidemic, the powers of the health department were significantly diminished, and its reputation in the city sank to an all-time low. This 1894 example serves to dramatize the relationship between politics and public health and to remind us that medical factors alone do not determine the course of public health events.

The 1894 smallpox epidemic in Milwaukee illustrates the dependence of nineteenth-century public health on political circumstances. Moreover, it shows that epidemics could have had—

Reprinted from Judith W. Leavitt, "Politics and Public Health," *Bull. History of Medicine*, 50 (1976): 553-568, by permission of The Johns Hopkins University Press. The research was aided in part by a Maurice L. Richardson Fellowship from the University of Wisconsin.

and occasionally did have—retrogressive as well as progressive effects on the development of the public health movement.

A frightening disease, with ugly physical manifestations, smallpox attacked all ages; exacerbated by unsanitary conditions and overcrowding, it spread quickly through a city. Victims who did not succumb to the disease were often left disfigured and pockmarked for life. But in the nineteenth century smallpox was a preventable disease since vaccination with cowpox virus was available. Thus one would not have expected it still to be a dreaded disease. However, although vaccination was quite widely used, it was not universally accepted in the medical community or among the lay public. Most medical practitioners advocated vaccination, but many thought it an inadequate protection against the disease; some anti-vaccinationists claimed it to be more harmful than the disease itself.[3]

Milwaukee newspapers aired the disagreements within the medical community over vaccination and about treatment of smallpox. The result was a confusion that seemed to grow as the century wore on. The presence of a large immigrant community in the city, among whom the efficacy of vaccination was most frequently questioned, merely increased dissension.[4]

The infrequent appearance of the disease and the confusion about medical theory account for a large part of the reaction Milwaukeeans had to smallpox. But the particular political circumstances that greeted the outbreak of an epidemic in the city also generated fear. Divided opinion among the people about how to react to the disease, and about whether or not to vaccinate occasionally sharpened already existing political and ethnic divisions in the city. In 1894 the Milwaukee Health Department found it difficult to control a medical situation because of its political ramifications.

Milwaukee in the 1890s was a bustling commercial and industrial city. Its population jumped from 20,000 at mid-century to 115,000 by 1880, and to 285,000 at the turn of the twentieth century. By 1910 Milwaukee was the twelfth largest city in the United States. Contrary to popular belief, its economy was based only partly on beer; other heavy and light industries also flourished.[5] Milwaukee contained members of almost every ethnic group that migrated to this country, with Germans and Poles predominating. Many have noted the German character of nineteenth-century Milwaukee.[6] Although most of its population lived in single-family, or two- to three-family dwellings, Milwaukee was very much an urban metropolis in the 1890s. Like all other cities in the United States during the period, it wrestled with the problems of housing congestion, street sanitation, and disposal of wastes.

In 1894 a Republican victory at the polls led to the appointment of a new health commissioner, Walter Kempster, a Republican and a nationally known psychiatrist. Although best known for his work with the insane, Kempster had spent much time studying how Europeans dealt with contagious diseases, especially cholera, and the new mayor felt that a man of such stature would be an asset to the city.[7]

The Milwaukee Common Council immediately questioned Kempster's appointment. Democrats might have been expected to oppose a Republican appointee as a matter of course; but Kempster's strongest opposition came from fellow Republicans, most vociferously from aldermen Robert Rudolph and Charles Kieckhefer, both representing German wards.[8] Both men criticized the fact that Kempster was new to Milwaukee and unfamiliar with the city and its problems. They opposed his appointment initially because they had supported other local physicians for the job. Kempster's English heritage and national reputation acted against him in the minds of those who sought a familiar, and possibly ethnic, representative of Milwaukee's population. But the majority of the council was willing to give Kempster a chance and confirmed his appointment by a vote of 23 to 13.[9]

With the nation and the city in the middle of a severe economic depression in 1894, the twenty-six patronage jobs controlled by the health commissioner assumed great significance. Although Kempster was a Republican, he was not susceptible to the influences of fellow party members. In fact, when he announced his appointees he completely ignored the party's suggested lists. Council members immediately challenged the appointments over which they had consent powers and vetoed some of them, establishing early the pattern that was to typify Kempster's relations with the legislative body.[10]

As a result of this episode, tension existed between the Health Department and the Common Council in June 1894 when the incidence of smallpox began to increase and an epidemic threatened. The atmosphere of cooperation necessary to cope successfully with an emergency situation was missing. Smallpox became the weapon with which certain members of the Common Council, led by southside saloon keeper Robert Rudolph, fought the health commissioner. The Polish and German immigrant groups most hard hit by the epidemic furnished the movement's political strength.

Dr. Kempster's reaction to smallpox in the city was similar to that of health commissioners before him. He at once hired extra physicians to launch a widespread vaccination campaign. He moved swiftly to isolate those patients reported to have the disease by removing them to the Isolation Hospital in the eleventh ward, acting under the 1892 ordinance giving him the power to do this forcibly if necessary. And he enforced a strict quarantine on those allowed to remain at home. The department also carried on extensive patient education campaigns and made wide use of the city's disinfecting van.[11]

The reaction of citizens to the Health Department's offensive was initially similar to the response during previous outbreaks. They cooperated with everything but vaccination, which the German and Polish areas of the city resisted. The health department had no authority to force vaccinations on anyone who did not want them, although non-vaccinated children could be refused admission to the public schools. Since the epidemic began just when the public schools were closing for the summer, this restraint was not particularly effective.[12]

During June and July smallpox appeared in all sections of the city, keeping the Health Department busy vaccinating and isolating reported cases. Kempster was confident that his procedures were effective and that an epidemic would not materialize. But by mid-July it was evident that a significant number of people were not cooperating with the health authorities. Many cases of smallpox went unreported. Discontent with the Health Department's policy grew when smallpox seemed to localize in the southside wards. The one hardest hit by the contagion was the eleventh ward, site of the Isolation Hospital and home of Alderman Rudolph.

At first Kempster denied that there was a seat of infection in the southside, but the numerous cases discovered there belied his assertions. Significant numbers of parents refused to allow their children to be examined or vaccinated by health officials, contributing to the rapid spread of the disease.[13] The immediate focus of the people's wrath was the Isolation Hospital in the crowded eleventh ward. Despite the renovations that had recently transformed the institution into what health authorities called a "modern facility," residents in the neighborhood still viewed it as a "pesthouse" and the source of their trouble. They claimed that it was a "menace to the health of citizens" and a "slaughterhouse" where patients "were not treated like human beings." Health officials maintained that the hospital was in good condition and offered good service to the poor who were admitted there.[14] Whatever the actual condition of the hospital in July and August 1894, southsiders were convinced that it was a death house for those who went there as patients and that its presence infected the nearby districts.[15]

A crisis was reached on August 5 when a crowd of neighbors successfully resisted an attempt by the health department to take a sick two-year-old child to the hospital. About 3,000 "furious" people armed with clubs, knives, and stones assembled in front of the child's house. The family had recently lost a child after it had been removed to the hospital, and the mother was frantic with fear and determined not to let the city "kill" (as she put it) another of her children. "I can give it better care and nourishment here than they can give it at the hospital. I will not allow my child to be taken to the hospital." Faced with the violent mob, and unable to control the situation, the ambulance on this occasion beat a hasty retreat.[16]

There is no evidence that Alderman Rudolph was in any way connected with the initial outburst on the night of August 5. But by the next day his name was being intimately linked with the southside "rioters," and he was participating actively to organize and mold the political force unleashed in his ward. On August 6 he introduced a resolution in the Common Council to remove the power of the health commissioner to take patients to the hospital against their will. Although the resolution had no effect against the ordinance that gave the power, its adoption was seen as a vote of support of the southsiders.[17] Rudolph appeared as a leader at public rallies. On August 7, when a crowd gathered to protest the night burial of a smallpox victim,

Rudolph addressed them with a speech that "was not entirely free from incendiarism." With his support, southsiders continued actively to protest health department activities.[18]

Dr. Kempster reacted by stiffening the official position, insisting that if smallpox spread it was not due to his department's negligence but rather to the rioters themselves spreading the contagion through the southside wards. He carefully defended every argument leveled at the department and told a reporter: "But for politics and bad beer, the matter would never have been heard of."[19] This belittlement of an issue as crucial as life itself to the southside residents did little to ease tensions between the Health Department and that section of the city. In fact, it emphasized the differences—class and ethnic—between Kempster and the immigrant southside residents. Showing little compassion, Kempster remained firm during the entire episode, never bending to the southsiders, never recognizing that their concerns may have been legitimate. "I am here to enforce the laws," he said, "and I shall enforce them if I have to break heads to do it. The question of the inhumanity of the laws I have nothing to do with."[20]

The situation on the southside clearly aided the spread of smallpox in that region of the city. Daily, crowds of people took to the streets, seeking out health officials to harrass. Quarantine officials keeping guard over houses were frequently the object of the mob's attack. With thousands of people roaming the streets and entering houses infected with smallpox, the contagion was destined to spread throughout the district. Case reports, despite the many concealed from authorities, indicate that the southside wards eleven and fourteen were most severely hit during the summer and fall of 1894.[21] (Figure 5-1)

The focus of the crowds' hatred was Dr. Kempster. He symbolized arbitrary governmental authority that was subverting immigrant culture and threatening personal liberty. Calling for his execution, crowds demanded that the "people's rights were paramount and should be protected, if need be, at the point of a pistol."[22] Women played a particularly important part in the disturbances. Since police were reluctant to use their clubs on "feminine shoulders," women were effective at maintaining disorder. Armed with clubs and stones, they assaulted the city police sent to preserve order. They threw stones and scalding

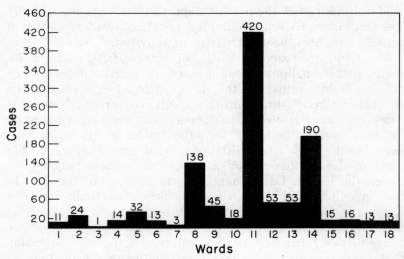

Figure 5-1. Milwaukee Smallpox Epidemic, 1894-1895, Ward Distribution. Wards 5, 11, 12, 14, and 17 were on the south side.

water at the ambulance horses in an effort to stop officials from removing any patients. As one newspaper observed the situation "Mobs of Pomeranian and Polish women armed with baseball bats, potato mashers, clubs, bed slats, salt and pepper, and butcher knives, lay in wait all day for . . . the Isolation Hospital van."[23]

City officials met daily to try to determine a course of action that would stem the riots and the spread of smallpox. They consulted the State Board of Health. Despite their efforts, the disturbances continued intermittently through August and into September.[24]

In addition to governmental meetings, southside citizen groups met to try to regain the image of that section as a peaceful place, safe for business. Deeply regretting "the notoriety which has been recently thrust upon that section of the city," one such meeting blamed the carelessness of the people for spreading the disease. Even the moderate groups, however, were not in sympathy with the Health Department; it was felt that the department had lost the confidence of the people and was thus no longer competent to deal with health emergencies.[25]

The activity in the eleventh ward diminished the effectiveness of the Health Department. Kempster himself admitted that although smallpox had been under control before the riots, quarantine was impossible and the spread of the disease inevitable since the mobs began roaming the streets.[26] Vaccinations, although freely available, were often rejected. During the violence on the south side the daily work of the Health Department virtually came to a halt. Patients could not be removed to the hospital in the face of weapon-wielding mobs, patients from other wards in the city could not be transported to the hospital through the hostile eleventh ward.[27] Kempster was denounced for attempting to remove patients to the hospital and further denounced when failure to remove such patients resulted in the spread of the epidemic. To a meeting of concerned physicians and businessmen, he voiced his frustrations:

> The laws are not enforced because the Common Council has prevented me. Not a single proposition that I have made . . . has been acted upon. . . . Proposition after proposition has been made to revise the laws as they now are. This has caused opposition among the people. We come to a house to remove a patient and are resisted. They tell us that their alderman informed them that next week the laws will be changed and they need not go. I have been tied hand and foot with investigations, injunctions and work that is never finished.[28]

At the beginning of September, with the opening of school, the coming of cooler weather, and increased police action against the rioters, the roving mobs on the southside became less visible. The focus of the anti-Kempster movement changed from street action to the Common Council as that body took up the battle in earnest.

Alderman Rudolph maintained a hold on his constituency and leadership of the mass movement against the Health Department by his actions and inflammatory rhetoric within the Common Council. There he introduced resolution after resolution and ordinance after ordinance, each one concerned with limiting the power of the Health Department and Walter Kempster. As a member of the Council Health Committee and as a close friend of the council's president, William G. Rauschenberger, Rudolph had considerable influence over health matters in the council.

Beginning with the measures introduced on August 6 to limit Kempster's powers to remove patients to the hospital, Rudolph's actions crescendoed as the epidemic itself increased in intensity. In early September he introduced an ordinance designed to accomplish what his earlier resolution could not: legally to tie the hands of the health commissioner by not allowing him to remove patients without their consent. The ordinance, revised slightly, passed the council and became law.[29]

Part of Rudolph's success in passing this ordinance was due to his scare tactics. The only member of the council in daily touch with the rioters, he promised renewed violence if the council did not pass his measure. He emoted loud and long on the injustices of tearing a child from its mother's breast, and he convinced his fellow politicians that voters would not be happy unless this measure passed. Council President Rauschenberger, who also thought Kempster incapable of handling the epidemic, actively supported Rudolph.[30]

In October, with the epidemic still raging about the city, Rudolph called for a special investigating committee to inquire into Kempster's activities, listing thirty-four charges against him.[31] The main charges were that Kempster had been negligent of his duties in the management of the Isolation Hospital, that he showed ignorance of quarantine methods, that patients were removed from their homes when they could have been better taken care of at their residences, and that the Health Department had grown tyrannical.[32] Twenty-eight physicians, including some of the more "prominent" physicians in the city, signed testimonials of misconduct on the part of the health commissioner.[33] Rudolph's charges were a serious matter.

Rudolph himself was appointed chairman of the council's committee to investigate the charges. The impeachment proceedings were front-page news in all the city's newspapers. Although most English-language papers declared that the investigation was a "farce" since it was led by so prejudiced a man, even the friendly *Sentinel* agreed that there was a need to clear the air.[34] The German-language press, on the other hand, endorsed Rudolph from the start and fully supported the impeachment proceedings.[35]

Rudolph's allies included the Anti-Vaccination Society, the German-language press, and the southside activists. There were many physicians among this group. Their leader was Dr. Emil Wahl, a German physician with a successful southside practice. Dr. Wahl was a member of the Milwaukee Medical Society (although he resigned from that organization when it accepted Kempster as a member), and his accusations that Kempster was incompetent to deal with the epidemic could not be dealt with lightly.[36]

There were genuine differences among physicians about the treatment of smallpox patients, as there had been on the vaccination issue. The division in the medical community was one between men of good faith, similarly trained, who used the tools of their profession to come to opposing conclusions. Dr. Wahl may or may not have been politically motivated to speak publicly against Dr. Kempster, but this does not necessarily mean that his medical disagreements were less real. His arguments were serious ones that the medical community seriously debated. Wahl's principle complaint was that Kempster was responsible for discharging patients from the hospital while they were still contagious, thus aiding the spread of the disease. The debate centered on the condition of the smallpox pustule at the various stages.

The epidemic reached its height during the month of October, when the impeachment hearings began. Southside physicians, led by Emil Wahl, gave testimony about patients who had been prematurely dismissed from the hospital. Kempster's cross-examination of these witnesses attempted to show their lack of familiarity with the disease and their inability to recognize its contagious states.[37] Witnesses also included southside families who felt wronged by the Health Department because it had attempted to remove their relatives to the hospital. It was claimed that Kempster had attempted to remove one patient who was not even ill with smallpox. A nurse who had served at the Isolation Hospital charged that the institution was mismanaged, that screens were not kept on the windows, and that its water supply was not adequate. In answering the charges against him, Kempster continued to deny any wrongdoing. The testimony of many leading physicians, including officers of the State Board of Health, supported him. The Milwaukee Medical Society also backed Kempster during the investigation. The health commissioner was obviously better able to withstand the public condemnations because of his medical colleague's approval.[38]

Judging that nine of the original thirty-four charges were sustained by the testimony, the investigation committee recommended conviction. Speculation ran high in the city about the council vote on the impeachment question, with newspapers predicting the decision. Daily shifts of various aldermen were front-page headlines. The council heard the relevant testimony for three days and nights consecutively. The exhausted aldermen were eager to be finished with the whole business. As the council neared the vote, its president complained: "I am at a loss to know whether we are attending a circus or a session of the Common Council." Excitement ran high, interruptions were frequent, and disorder was rampant. Finally, in February 1895, with the epidemic not yet over, the council voted 22 to 14 to dismiss the health commissioner.[39]

Although the impeachment vote did not divide along party lines, the move against Kempster was nonetheless political. Patronage, class, and ethnic divisions were responsible for a significant part of the opposition to Kempster in the city. Physicians who sought his post or appointments within the Health Department were disappointed and resentful of the man who held office, and Republican politicians were bitter because of their loss of influence in department appointments.[40] From the beginning of his tenure in office, Kempster had labored against a vocal opposition. When the epidemic struck the city, the opposition had a weapon to use to successfully resist the health officer. The issue of the Isolation Hospital was one that carried with it a tradition of anxiety and fear and was easily employed to gather support against Kempster. The issue of forcible removal of children from their homes was one that pulled at the heartstring of every immigrant parent. The *Sentinel* termed the movement against Kempster a "cabal." Although it might be hard to document such a conspiracy, there is no question that Kempster's position in Milwaukee, while it may have been medically sound, was politically untenable. He had few friends and many enemies on the Common Council.[41]

Ethnic divisions in the city were evident from the differences in reactions between the English-language papers that supported Kempster and the German-language press that rejoiced over his dismissal.[42] Analysis of the impeachment vote shows that the ethnic divisions within the city held. Those wards that contained large numbers of German and Polish immigrants, or their descendents, were those that sustained the impeachment vote. Those wards that were largely populated by American-born or by immigrant groups other than German and Polish, voted for Kempster. Party affiliations did not determine the vote, since both Democrats and Republicans on the council were split. Figure 5-2 illustrates the close correlation between German and Polish ethnicity and the vote against Kempster.[43]

The smallpox epidemic of 1894 severely divided the city of Milwaukee, causing political conflicts and resentments that were long-lived. Most significantly for our interest, it had a retrogressive effect on public health in Milwaukee. Traditionally epidemics were times when health authorities increased their powers. This had been true in Milwaukee and in other American cities. In 1894 in Milwaukee the opposite happened. During the height of the epidemic, with fear running high, the council repealed those health measures that were seen as effective in halting the spread of the disease and fired the physician who supported those techniques. As Figure 5-3 illustrates, the moves against Kempster were all initiated while the epidemic was still raging in the city. Within the space of the ten months from May 1894, when Dr. Kempster took office, to February 1895, when he was dismissed, the Common Council deprived the Health Department of some of the powers important for it to be effective, and ultimately deprived the health commissioner of his job. Kempster appealed the impeachment decision and was reinstated as health commissioner after one year. The episode,

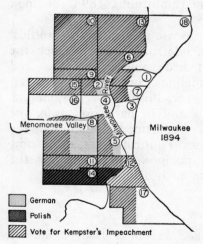

Figure 5-2. Ethnic Vote for Kempster's Impeachment.

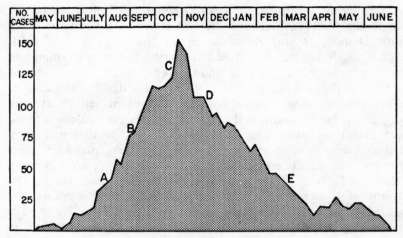

REPORTED CASES

Figure 5-3. Milwaukee Smallpox Epidemic, 1894-1895, Reported Cases and Moves against Kempster.
A. August 6, 1894. Resolution on forcible removal.
B. September 4, 1894. Ordinance on forcible removal.
C. October 15, 1894. Resolution for impeachment investigation; revised ordinance on forcible removal.
D. November 26, 1894. Revised ordinance on forcible removal passed.
E. February 21, 1895. Common Council impeaches Health Commissioner.

however, affected the Health Department permanently. It never regained powers lost during the tumultuous 1894 smallpox epidemic.[44]

Milwaukee's history with the disease illustrates the political nature of the issue of smallpox control. Slowly through the century the Health Department had gained confidence and control over the treatment of smallpox, until by 1894 it felt secure in its powers. But in that year, during a severe epidemic, the Common Council challenged and in part took away the most traditional of all Health Department functions: the ability to control epidemic diseases. Political issues, only some of which were directly related to smallpox, determined how the municipal government handled the medical emergency.

Notes

1. Charles Rosenberg, studying the effects of cholera epidemics on American cities, noted: "The cholera epidemics of the nineteenth century provided much of the impetus needed to overcome centuries of governmental inertia and indifference in regard to problems of public

health. . . . It is not surprising that the growing public health movement found in cholera an effective ally," *The Cholera Years: The United States in 1832, 1849, and 1866* [Chicago: University of Chicago Press 1962], pp. 2-3. See also John Duffy, who posits that cholera and yellow fever were "important factors in promoting public health measures," because of their "crisis" presentation ("The Social Impact of Disease in the Late Nineteenth Century," *Bulletin of the New York Academy of Medicine* 47 [1971]:800. Although Duffy saw smallpox running a poor third to cholera and yellow fever, in Milwaukee smallpox took the place of the former two diseases, which did not threaten the city after 1850. The parallel with cholera and yellow fever is drawn despite the major differences between those diseases and smallpox, the availability of a preventative for one and not the others. While vaccination raises interesting differences between the examples used here, those differences did not affect the public reaction evoked in each case: fear and panic and an immediate governmental response to alleviate conditions.

2. Smallpox first appeared in Milwaukee in 1843 and reappeared three years later in virulent form. A major epidemic occurred in 1868 immediately after the Board of Health was established, and was responsible for establishing certain power patterns that were to remain throughout the century. During the 1870s Milwaukee suffered two major outbreaks of smallpox. Despite the fact that smallpox was never a major cause of death in Milwaukee, it aroused more interest on the part of the public authorities and was responsible for more public health legislation than any other disease.

3. See Martin Kaufman, "The American Anti-vaccinationists and their Arguments," *Bulletin of the History of Medicine* 41 (1967): 463-78. Kaufman describes most anti-vaccinationists as irregular practioners and identifies the movement with sectarian medicine. It is not clear to me that division holds in Milwaukee, where many regularly trained physicians were hesitant about the protective value of vaccination throughout the nineteenth century.

4. Ibid., p. 474, Kaufman also noticed the prevalence of strong anti-vaccinationist sentiment among the immigrants, specifically the German immigrants. Not only were immigrants in Milwaukee vocal against vaccination, but other governmental health services drew their wrath. Placarding a home containing an infectious disease, removing sick to an isolation hospital, requiring private night burials, were all seen by newly arrived Germans and Poles as direct infringements on their personal liberties and were vigorously resisted in Milwaukee. For more on this reaction of Milwaukee immigrants, see Judith Walzer Leavitt, "Public Health in Milwaukee 1867-1910" (Ph. D. diss., University of Chicago, 1975). The reaction was found throughout the state of Wisconsin. See for example, the *Sixth Annual Report of the State Board of Health of Wisconsin, 1881,* pp. 116, 120; and the *Fifteenth Annual Report of the State Board of Health of Wisconsin, 1894-1895* pp. 138-39, 163.

5. For more on Milwaukee's economy see Byard Still, *Milwaukee: The History of a City* (Madison: State Historical Society of Wisconsin, 1965) and Roger David Simon, "The Expansion of an Industrial City: Milwaukee, 1880-1910," (Ph.D diss., University of Wisconsin, 1971).

6. On the German population of Milwaukee and its assimilation, see Gerd Korman, *Industrialization, Immigrants and Americanizers: The View from Milwaukee 1866-1921* (Madison: State Historical Society 1967) and Kathleen Neils Conzen, "The German Athens: Milwaukee and the Accomodation of its Immigrants 1836-1860," (Ph.D diss., University of Wisconsin, 1972).

7. Walter Kempster had only small ties of any kind to the city of Milwaukee. He had a national reputation as a physician to the insane and had held posts at the State Lunatic Asylum at Utica, New York, and the Northern Hospital for the Insane at Oshkosh, Wisconsin. He had testified for the prosecution in the Guiteau case. He had moved to Milwaukee in 1890 but since that time had been on two missions abroad studying cholera and investigating Jewish emigration from Russia. His tenure in the city of Milwaukee, his critics were quick to point out, had been short indeed. For biographical material on Walter Kempster, see the *Dictionary of American Biography* (New York: Charles Scribner's Sons, 1933) 324-25; Howard Kelly and Walter Burrage, *American Medical Biographies*, (Baltimore: Norman, Remington Co., 1920), pp. 652-53; and most throughly, F. M. Sperry, *A Group of Distinguished Physicians and Surgeons of Milwaukee* (Chicago: J. H. Beers & Co. 1904), pp. 56-69. See also Kempster's obituary, *Milwaukee Sentinel,* 23 August 1918, and *New York Times*, 23 August 1918, p. 9. Kempster was buried in Arlington National Cemetery.

8. *Milwaukee Sentinel,* 17, 18, 24, 30, April 1894.

9. Eight Republicans opposed and five Democrats supported Kempster. Without Democratic support, the Republican nominee would not have been confirmed. *Common Council Proceedings,* 30 April 1894. See also the *Milwaukee Sentinel,* 1 May 1894.

10. *Milwaukee Sentinel,* 12, 26, June 1894; *Common Council Proceedings,* 11 June 1894, p. 32, 14 May 1894, p. 61.

11. *Seventeenth Annual Report of the Milwaukee Health Department, 1894,* pp. 26-32; *Eighteenth Annual Report of the Milwaukee Health Department, 1895,* pp. 10-12. *Eighteenth and Nineteenth Annual Report of the Health Department, 1895* pp. 35-39. *Milwaukee Sentinel,* 28 June, 4 July 1894. Physicians were urged to cooperate with health officials in reporting the disease. The health commissioner closed schools when he thought necessary. See the *Milwaukee Sentinel,* 2, 3 September; 3, 13, 24 November 1894. See also the *School Board Proceedings,* Milwaukee, 6 November 1894, pp. 124-125.

12. At least two German language newspapers argued that vaccination did not protect against smallpox and that its effects were often worse than the disease it was to prevent. The Anti-Vaccination Society disseminated its information through pamphlets widely circulated in three languages. *Milwaukee Sentinel,* 1 August 1894.

13. *Milwaukee Sentinel,* 23 July 1894. See also 24 July 1894.

14. *Milwaukee Sentinel,* 3, 4, 6 August 1894. The anti-hospital sentiment expressed by residents of the south side reopened a familar Milwaukee debate about moving the hospital outside the city limits. The issue flared up, encompassed much time for the city's legal staff, and was

finally dropped at the end of the summer. Most physicians were against removal from the city limits, as long distance travel was not seen as beneficial to an acutely ill patient, nor was it convenient for physicians.

15. The theory of air-born contagion is not yet disproved as one way in which the smallpox virus might travel. It has also been shown that flies have acted as vectors in spreading the disease. See Cyril W. Dixon, *"Smallpox* (London J & A Churchill, 1962), p. 264. This theory was supported at the time because the eleventh ward was in fact the main seat of infection in the city. Certainly popular opinion very strongly blamed the Isolation Hospital for the large number of smallpox cases on the south side. See the *Milwaukee Sentinel,* 4 August 1894.

16. The mother is quoted in the *Milwaukee Sentinel,* 6 August 1894. For more on the episode, see the *Eighteenth and Nineteenth Annual Report of the Milwaukee Health Department, 1895* pp. 42-43. For a brief popularized account of the riots, see Richard L. Stefanik, "The smallpox riots of 1894," *Historical Messenger,* December 1970, pp. 123-28.

17. *Common Council Proceedings,* 6 August 1894, p. 326. See also the *Milwaukee Sentinel,* 7 August 1894; and the *Eighteenth and Nineteenth Annual Report for the Milwaukee Health Department,* 1895, pp. 41-42. The initial ordinance had been passed in reaction to a cholera scare in the city in 1892 and had never been used.

18. For more on the August 7 rally, see the *Milwaukee Daily News,* a workingman's newspaper, which tended to support the rioters but not the riots in early August. "There is reason to believe that there has been some basis for the many criticisms . . . made" (8 August 1894). The *Sentinel,* however, was quick to blame the "ignorance of the people" in not following existing health regulations and in defying authorities. (8 August 1894).

19. *Milwaukee Sentinel,* 7 August 1894.

20. Quoted in the *Milwaukee Daily News,* 11 August 1894.

21. Out of a total of 1,074 cases, 846 were from the south side wards— half of these were from the eleventh ward.

22. *Milwaukee Sentinel,* 9 August 1894.

23. *Milwaukee Sentinel,* 30 August 1894. For more on the role of women in the rioting, see the *Sentinel* 10, 12, August 1894; and the *Milwaukee Daily News,* 10 August 1894.

24. For details about the involvement of the State Board of Health see the *Wisconsin State Board of Health Report,* 1893-1894, "Report of the Executive Committee Relative to the Smallpox Situation in the City of Milwaukee," pp. 56-69; U.O.B. Wingate, "Smallpox in Wisconsin from January 1894 to June 1895," *Public Health : Papers and Reports of the American Public Health Association* 1896, 21:268-72; the *Eighteenth and Nineteenth Annual Report of the Milwaukee Health Department,* 1895 pp. 49-58; and the *Milwaukee Sentinel,* 11, 12, 14, August 1894.

25. *Milwaukee Sentinel,* 12, 14, August 1894.

26. *Milwaukee Sentinel,* 12 August 1894.

27. *Evening Wisconsin,* 29 August 1894.

28. Quoted in the *Sentinel,* 23 October 1894.

29. *Common Council Proceedings,* Milwaukee, 4 September, 1 Oct-

ober, 26 November 1894. See a copy of the ordinance as passed in the Appendix to the 1894-1895 *Proceedings*, pp. 22-23. Section provided: "The commissioner of health shall not remove to any Isolation Hospital in said city any child or person suffering from any disease who can be nursed and cared for during such illness in his or her home during the continuance of the disease except upon the recommendation and advice of the said commissioner of health or one of the assistant commissioners of health, and the physician, if any, attending upon such child or person, not being a member of the health department of said city; and in case such commissioner or assistant commissioner, and such physician shall be unable to agree as to the advisability of removing such child or person, then they shall call in and appoint another physician not a member of the health department, and the decision of the majority of such physicians and commissioners or assistant commissioner shall be decisive of the question. The third physician called in, as above provided, shall not receive or be entitled to any fees from the city for consultation of service in the decision of the case submitted to such board of physicians." The conditions were so burdensome they effectively tied the hands of a health commissioner attempting to act swiftly to stem an epidemic.

30. *Milwaukee Sentinel*, 4, 5 September; 2, 6, 7, 9 October, 2 December 1894; *Evening Wisconsin*, 8 October 1894. See also *Eighteenth and Nineteenth Annual Report to the Milwaukee Health Department, 1895*, p. 69; and the *Common Council Proceedings*, 4 September 1894.

31. *Common Council Proceedings*, 15 October 1894, pp. 524-531. Although the two actions discussed here, ordinances for the removal of patients and impeachment, were not the only ones Alderman Rudolph initiated against the health commissioner, they were the most important and thus form the focus of the discussion here. For additional measures that the Council considered at Rudolph's initiation, see *Common Council Proceedings*, 20 August 1894, pp. 364-365.; 4 September 1894, pp. 374-75; 15 October 1894, p. 497; 29 October 1894, p. 571; 12 November 1894, p. 583. See also the *Milwaukee Sentinel* 21 August, 1 September, 2, 13 October 1894.

32. *Milwaukee Sentinel*, 16 October 1894.

33. Of the 28, at least 19 were members of the local medical society, the Wisconsin State Medical Society, or the American Medical Association. See the membership list of the Milwaukee Medical Society and the local AMA members in the archives of the Milwaukee Academy of Medicine. The membership list of the State Medical Society was in the *Wisconsin Medical Journal*, 1903-1904, pp. 196-208. At least two of the physicians had been brought to court by Kempster, charged with not reporting smallpox, which might account for their hostile position.

34. See the *Milwaukee Sentinel, Milwaukee Daily News*, and *Evening Wisconsin, passim*, 15 October 1894, to 21 February 1895. See for example editorial of 5 January 1895, in the *Sentinel* entitled "The Farce Continued." Other newspapers voiced similar sentiments. The *Milwaukee Catholic Citizen* ridiculed the matter of putting the "prosecuting attorney on the bench as the judge of the case" (20 October 1894).

35. See, for example, *Seebote* and *Herold, passim*, in these months.

36. For biographical material on Emil Wahl, see Louis Frank *The Medical History of Milwaukee 1834-1914.* (Milwaukee: Germania Press 1915), p. 72. He appears on the membership list of the Milwaukee Medical Society, having joined the organization in 1888. For more on Wahl's resignation, see the Milwaukee Medical Society minutes, 22 January 1895 and 12 February 1895, in the archives of the Milwaukee Academy of Medicine.

37. *Milwaukee Sentinel,* 15, 16, 17, 28, 29, November, 4, 5, December 1894; 4-16 January 1895. See also the *Milwaukee Journal,* 4-10 January 1895.

38. At a joint meeting, medical society members and business leaders hissed Rudolph's name while loudly cheering Kempster's. See the *Sentinel,* 23 October 1894. The transcripts of the impeachment proceedings are unfortunately lost and it is impossible to discern the technical aspects of the medical debate from the newspaper accounts.

39. For the press assessment of how the vote would be, see the *Sentinel,* 14, 15, 16, 18, February 1895; *Journal,* 18 February 1895; and the *Daily News,* 18, February 1895. See a description to the final session in the *Journal,* 21 February 1895; *Sentinel,* 21 February 1895.

40. For contemporary arguments along these lines, see the *Milwaukee Sentinel,* 30, 31, August, 2, 4, September 1894; 20, 22, February 1895; 21 January 1896; *Daily News,* 31 August 1894; *Journal,* 19 February 1895; *Catholic Citizen,* 8 September 1894.

41. *Milwaukee Sentinel,* 22 February 1895.

42. See, for example, the editorial in the *Herold,* 22 February 1895, in which it noted: "The decision of the Common Council . . . will be received by the great majority of the population with satisfaction. It is the confirmation of many months experience and the conviction that [Kempster] is not the right man to execute those measures necessary in the case of an epidemic. . . . [He] is not master of the situation and could not awaken the general trust which is, after all, in such a case, a necessary prerequisite." I am grateful to Edith Hoshino Altbach for help in translating this editorial.

43. The sources of ethnicity were the *Eleventh United States Census,* 1890, and the *Wisconsin State Census.* Precise population figures were not available by ward.

44. See the *Sentinel,* 18 January 1896. For a copy of the judge's decision, see the *Eighteenth and Nineteenth Annual Report,* 1895, pp. 81-85.

PART III

CHARITY, SCIENCE, AND CLASS: THE INSTITUTIONS OF MEDICINE

The contemporary awareness of our massive societal investment in health care has engendered a debate over what services should be provided and how the health system should be structured. Furthermore, there has been a reevaluation of the goals and responsibilities of health institutions. The following articles examine the economic, political, and intellectual climate that shaped and transformed asylums, hospitals, and medical schools in the nineteenth and early twentieth centuries.

Morris J. Vogel examines the wide-ranging implications for patients and physicians of the transformation of the hospital from a welfare to a medical institution. David Rosner weighs the implications of a crisis in hospital financing for the institutions' internal governance, control, and function. In particular, he focuses on the resultant changing services for working-class patients. Richard Brown investigates the growing role of foundations in American medicine after 1910. He is specifically concerned with the stormy relationship between medical educators and foundations over the introduction of full-time clinical professorships. Barbara Rosenkrantz and Maris Vinovskis compare two pre-Civil War mental asylums. They analyze how the growing concern of hospital superintendents with their statistics affected their understanding of death and responsibility for life.

All of these essays look at the dynamics of social change and the internal developments in medical institutions. Further questions remain to be answered. Who defines the goals and policies of medical institutions? How is the hospital's charity and welfare function transformed with the growing importance of medical science? Is this function lost or does it take on new forms? As the site of health care delivery shifts from the family to the hospital, how does this affect different household members and families from different classes? How do changing conceptions of the medical system's responsibility for death shape medical care at different moments in history? Why do outside forces play a greater role in shaping health care institutions at particular moments in time?

6 The Transformation of the American Hospital, 1850-1920

In the beginning—and for the American general hospital the beginning extends into the middle of the nineteenth century—the hospital was a largely undifferentiated welfare institution. Its patients were socially marginal, overwhelmingly poor, and often without roots in the community. In cities with substantial immigrant populations—Boston, New York, Philadelphia—the majority of hospital patients was likely to be foreign-born in any year during the second half of the nineteenth century. The majority of expectant mothers who entered lying-in hosptials in northeastern cities in the period were generally confined for illegitimate births. Dependence as much as disease still distinguished hospital patients from the public at large.[1] To most Americans the hospital was an alien institution.

There was little medical reason for patients to enter a hospital. There were also strong cultural biases against hospitalization. In case of illness most Americans did not seek the advice of a physician but relied either on self-dosing and other home remedies or on a greater tolerance for and acceptance of affliction.[2] Most who sought the care of a doctor expected that medical treatment would take place within the boundaries of everyday experience. Physicians kept track of their seriously ill patients with frequent home visits, and even the most difficult surgical procedures were performed in the home, often in the kitchen. Accident victims were even taken to their homes for care.[3] City dwellers too poor to afford medical fees might secure—either on an out-patient basis or in their own homes—the gratuitous services of a dispensary physician or surgeon. Sickness was generally endured in its traditional setting, in the home and among family.

History stigmatized the hospital. It had evolved from the almshouse and pesthouse, institutions in which the welfare of the patient was often secondary to the well-being of the society that required his isolation.[4] Further, hospital care in the pre-antiseptic age might be life-threatening. Sepsis, infection, was often called hospitalism, a rhetorical tribute to the institution.

The hospital posed other difficulties for mid-nineteenth century medicine. Because therapeutic intervention was of only limited efficacy, much of medical practice consisted of environmental manipulation. The role of the physician was not limited to narrowly technical, physiologically oriented remedies. The physician had to understand the patient's social ecology and his constitution; ideally, he offered advice and treatment appropriate for the contexts within which the patient lived and worked. In the terminology of the mid-nineteenth century, as well as our own, medical practice was family oriented.[5] Treating a patient in the hospital meant treating an abstraction.

Yet there were patients for the more than one hundred hospitals that existed by 1873.[6] These patients were predominantly the desperate, victims of a catalog of social ills and personal failings. Treatment and care were acts of charity. The great majority of American general hospitals, then as now, were voluntary organizations. In the nineteenth century they were supported by the philanthropy of the wealthy that mixed self-interest and genuine social concern. By shouldering the burdens of and maintaining a genuine pietistic belief in the stewardship role, philanthropists justified class distinctions. Although hospital donors displayed self-interest in making their contributions— advancing their visions of a harmonious social order and advancing the careers of the hospital practitioners with whom they often shared intimate social ties—donors did not expect that they or their families would ever be likely to use the hospital.

Given the nature of the patient population, the orientation of medical practice, and the social attitudes of donors, the hospital regimen of the mid-nineteenth century is not surprising. Both medicine and charity rationalized, justified, and required the same sort of treatment: Patients were to be treated as moral beings. To secure admission a prospective patient often had to bring a written statement from a morally, socially, or economically significant person, testifying to the applicant's good character.[7] To gain admission as a free patient—the only possibility for someone too poor to pay the two weeks board in advance required by the Massachusetts General Hospital and other hospitals in 1870—required sponsorship by a hospital donor, or at least the approval of a committee of the lay trustees. There was no alternative to the free bed for the hospital's patient constituency. At the Massachusetts General Hospital in 1870 there was an average patient census of 120 and an average free bed census of 89.[8] Finally, lay trustees controlled hospital admissions until the second half of the nineteenth century. Thus, for many years laymen actually determined whom to admit.

The moral nature of the admissions process being what it was, the hospital was not simply or primarily an agency of social control. The admissions process often worked to exclude the potentially deviant, those from whom society thought it had the most to fear. At Massachusetts General in the mid-nineteenth century, the Irish—swelling the city's population and threatening its stability—were largely excluded.[9] The admission of blacks was generally restricted for much of the century.

The paternalism of the admissions process was duplicated in the treatment accorded patients within the hospital's walls. The word walls is used advisedly. During the course of the mid-nineteenth century one can discern a sort of competition among hospitals to wall themselves in. Masonry walls replaced picket fences around hospital grounds. Annual reports pointed proudly to impermiable eight-foot structures.[10] The nature of the hospital's patients brought about the building of walls. The nineteenth-century patient was not the bedridden, acute-care case of the modern hospital but was often quite ambulatory. Walls and guarded gates enabled institutions to control the comings and goings of the institutionalized. A patient needed a signed pass to spend the day in the city.

In addition, until late in the nineteenth century hospital patients were often new to the city and to the discipline of an urban and industrial society. Throughout the 1870s, for example, fewer than 10 percent of patients at the Massachusetts General Hospital were born in Boston. Those who controlled the institution felt they could never be quite sure of the behavior of their charges. Hospital walls served to isolate hospital patients in a paternalistic, authoritarian environment. The high masonry wall cut patients off from intercourse with outsiders so that alcohol and tobacco could not be introduced into the hospital. Along the same lines, family and friends visiting patients were sometimes searched for contraband before entry. Visiting hours themselves were severely restricted. It was not uncommon to limit patients to one visitor per day and to limit visiting to one inconvenient hour in the middle of the working day, closing off the hospital altogether on Sundays. Children's Hospital in Boston allowed one relative at a time between 11 and 12 o'clock on Monday, Wednesday, and Friday mornings. At the same time, hospital donors from whom there was no fear of moral contagion, were invited to visit patients at any time and to participate in the moral/medical healing process through encouraging patients "by word or counsel."[11] Patients were expected to behave themselves; rude language was forbidden, as was card playing. When physicians made ward visits, patients were to sit up silently in bed. The ultimate punishment for patient misbehavior was expulsion from the hospital.[12]

The hospital patient, at least until the last quarter of the nineteenth century, was therefore stigmatized as dependent and somehow unworthy. The hospital figured prominently in the almost chronic discussion of "charity abuse," the code phrase in the mid-nineteenth century for the conviction that promiscuous charity sapped the moral will of its recipients and left them unable to look after themselves. Medical abuse was the hospital version of this complaint. While a majority of the charitably inclined probably considered sickness and accident a sufficient means test of the sincerity and worthiness of the hospital patient, it is fairly easy to pick out of the discussion of medical abuse the lurking suspicion that patients were perversely and deliberately coming down with pneumonia or being crushed by collapsing excavations in order to gain entrance to the hospital.[13]

The phrase "charitable institution," when applied to the nineteenth-century hospital, means a great deal more, then, than a place that dispensed free medical care. Paternalism and authoritarianism greeted the hospital patient. The humane feelings of the social elite who supported and managed the hospital, and the medical elite who served it, were diminished by the cultural and social distance that divided hospital patient from patron and practitioner. It was within this context that the order and control necessary for the functioning of the hospital were instituted.

Practitioners, no less than patients, played their role in the nineteenth-century drama of hospital charity. The minority of physicians who practiced in hospitals did so gratuitously. Though hospital patients generally paid no fees and hospitals did not salary medical attendants, a hospital position enabled a medical man to see and treat numbers of special cases (comparatively rare in private practice) and so develop a reputation that would itself be remunerative. Hospital physicians earned their livelihoods by caring for well-to-do private patients who paid for the physician's knowledge gained in hospital work. Private practice remained the norm. Although the nineteenth-century hospital was not the center of the doctor's work world, the few hours he put in there each day, during his term of perhaps three months each year, did not represent income lost. Boston's Dr. Henry J. Bigelow noted in 1889 that hospital connections offered "certain well-understood advantages"; unpaid "hospital offices would command a considerable premium in money from the best class of practitioners were they annually put up at auction."[14] This attractiveness did not derive alone from the prospect of increased earnings. Such a prospect was linked to the style of practice that a hospital or dispensary affiliation might be expected to generate. A report of the Boston Dispensary suggested the interrelatedness of material and psychic rewards:

> It is not to be supposed that the motives of the attending physicians have been wholly foreign from considerations of personal advantage. They have doubtless been actuated by the hope of professional improvement and the prospect of building up an honest fame, as well as by the desires of fulfilling the benevolent intuitions of this charity.[15]

Hospital practitioners were not a cross-section of the medical profession. Henry J. Bigelow, Boston's leading surgeon, spoke in 1871 of the "two classes of the profession," differentiating those who simply practiced medicine from those who contributed to its development.[16] This latter group was the medical elite; in eastern cities this group benefited from—and defined itself, in part, in terms of—hospital and dispensary experience.

The medical elite was to some measure a product of social background. Bigelow probably would not have included all illustriously connected practitioners in his higher class of the profession, but family background was more than an indicator of medical status. Family background opened certain options. The upper-class medical graduate of the nineteenth century had the means to delay practice and to pursue European study after obtaining his American degree, if he were so inclined. Further, the properly connected young physician might be motivated to choose the European education that distinguished the best medical work in America. The fortunes of birth and family and class expectation encouraged him to view his career as more than a nasty struggle for economic success.

The good intentions and professional aspirations of hospital practitioners were not universally applauded. To the great mass of the profession, patients treated gratuitously in the hospital represented income lost to non-hospital practitioners. While hospital patients were overwhelmingly the poor, those whose funds were too limited to pay medical fees, this problem was minimal. But as the middle class increasingly resorted to the hospital in the late nineteenth century, the problem grew more serious and the debate more shrill. By 1909 the Boston Medical Society was complaining about the "rising feeling" that surgery could be performed only in hospitals, "thus depriving all ordinary private physicians and surgeons of a class of cases." The society condemned the city's hospitals for "inculcating in the minds of the laity a lack of confidence in the abilities of the ordinary private practitioner."[17]

By the turn of the century medical and social forces alike led to the use of the hospital by the middle classes. The bachelor movement noted by contemporaries—that is, the dramatically increased tendency of young middle-class adults to move away from their families and take up housekeeping on their own until married, if they married at all—resulted in numbers of relatively affluent individuals without families to care for them in illness.[18] This growing dependence on hospitals by young adults was matched at the other end of the age spectrum by the survival of greater numbers of individuals into old age, often also without families or proper homes for care in illness, even though they might be relatively affluent.

Changes in urban living patterns also meant that those who continued to live within family structures, often found themselves in smaller homes or apartments without the requisite spatial amenities for the care of the sick. Finally, as Talcott Parsons and Renée Fox note, "the special character of the American urban family" (and they mean the modern middle-class family), "which is extremely vulnerable to certain types of strain," leads to an increased reliance on the hospital. They characterize this family by its small size, its apparant lack of economic function, and its isolation, as a conjugal family, from other elements of the kinship system. As the scope of the family's activities have narrowed, Parsons and Fox note, the emotional significance of the relationships within it have increased, thus saddling members with a heavy burden from which sickness offers an escape. But a sickness suffered in the home by a family member upsets a precariously balanced, emotionally charged family system, thus harming the family, as well as retarding the cure of the sick person. Therapy, then, they argue "is more easily effected in a professional milieu, when there is not the same order of intensive emotional involvement so characteristic of family relationships."[19] The psychic and emotional burdens of a sickness suffered in the home were not missed by contemporaries. A turn-of-the-century Boston City Hospital report noted that the return of the still helpless sick to their homes would "add to the domestic burdens of a family already struggling under difficulties to maintain itself."[20] No social factors could have made the hospital a viable alternative for the middle classes during sickness, however, without the conquest of hospital infection made possible in the last quarter of the century by antisepsis and then asepsis.

Changes in medical perception and therapeutics also led more directly to the hospitalization of the non-poor. The closing years of the century began to witness the evolution of a range of diagnostic advances and specific therapeutic regimens that fostered an increasingly dominant view of the body as a mechanism and a lessening commitment to understanding the patient as a social organism.[21] Germ theory and the expansion of surgery recast medicine's perception of patients; no longer would they need to be treated within their social context. At the same time that the medical necessity for home treatment diminished, the hospital offered convenience and a likely setting for the more technical and narrow practice of medicine that was beginning to emerge by century's end. As the institution that had made specialization possible, it offered a site in which specialization could follow its own logic. Ultimately, the hospital would also be able to concentrate within its walls the newly developing complex technology of medicine. By the 1920s medical and surgical (but not obstetrical) patients at urban hospitals nearly represented cross-sections of their communities.[22]

As the hospital became more attractive to the middle classes, its identification with the poor diminished. This change in the social nature of the patient class was partly responsible for the relaxation of the institution's moralistic posture. Contributing to this also, of course, was the fact that medicine itself, as it grew ever more narrow and technical, increasingly divorced itself from its traditional moral concerns. Finally, the fact that hospital patients themselves were sicker (they would rarely be in the institution because of dependence by the end of the century) would have made it more difficult to manipulate them socially and morally, were anyone so inclined. This is not to say that the institution developed a completely humane attitude toward the patient. Medical absolutism supplanted the charity mentality in discomfitting the hospital patient.[23]

The more serious nature of the hospital patients' illnesses and the increasingly scientific and technical orientation of medicine (and these are interrelated phenomena) introduce the last element in the transformation of the institution to be discussed here: expense. Simply stated, perhaps exaggerated, it cost more to take care of sick people than to look after tired, or hungry, or homeless individuals. In 1870 operating expenses at the Massachusets General Hospital were $62,800. By 1910 they had reached $350,300. The average cost per patient per week mounted from $10.04 in 1870 to $25.15 in 1910 and to $39.90 in 1920.[24] This rise in costs can also be demonstrated anecdotally by looking at examples in which individuals and institutions did not understand, or did not sympathize with, the level of expenditure necessary to operate the "new hospital."

Dr. Thomas Howell of Worcester, Massachusetts, was such a traditionalist. Physicians who trained at hospitals equipped with modern paraphernalia, he noted, would be handicapped when they had to adjust to private practice:

Not having been taught to improvise, they do not realize how much can be accomplished with the crude implements to be found in the ordinary household. The graduates of cheaply equipped institutions, on the other hand, have been required to exercise ingenuity throughout their apprenticeship, and, as a result, they are not only more resourceful in emergencies, but their adaptability enhances their professional reputation.

Asepsis provided excuses for the most lavish expenditures of all. These costs were obviously unnecessary. Did not mortality rates from home surgery compare favorably to those of the most lavishly equipped operating rooms?[25]

To some accustomed to medicine as it had been and the tradition of the hospital as a charity, the hospital's new requirements fell into the category of extravagance. George Ludlam, lay superintendent of the New York Hospital and president of the American Hospital Association in 1906, commented on the difficulty of working with doctors trained in scientific medicine: "Familiarity with these methods engenders a spirit of extravagance which permeates the whole establishment and which it is exceedingly difficult to check or control." Wedded to the concept of the hospital as a charity, Ludlam made a fetish of controlling expenses. He was proud of New York Hospital's answer to the spiraling cost of maintaining a medical library: "I am absolutely at a loss for an understanding of the value of a medical library in a hospital," he announced as his hospital shut its library, gave away its books, and put the space to better use as a nurses' reception room. Ludlam saved his most righteous indignation for the rubber gloves then becoming a necessary condition for maintaining asepsis:

There has grown up in the hospital with which I am connected, a custom which I do not think I characterize by any exaggerated expression when I call it a craze for the use of rubber gloves. Beginning in a small way, our consumption of that item has increased from year to year until, absolutely and positively, I should be ashamed to tell you what we spent for rubber gloves last year. I go to our attending staff and call their attention to it. They say it is deplorable, but rubber gloves have come to be a very important item in the treatment of surgical cases. . . . I went to one doctor recently, and said, "Doctor, I notice that all your assistants now in the operating theatre, even down to the orderlies, are wearing rubber gloves at the operation. I notice that the house staff in their ordinary attention to the patients in the ward making ordinary ward dressings and the nurses who attend them are all wearing rubber gloves. Now is this last necessary?" . . . "Oh, no [they respond] , it is far more important to use rubber gloves in the ward dressing than in the operating department."[26]

In a milder way, the Massachusetts General Hospital trustees shared this same bewilderment at the mounting financial demands made by modern medicine. Upset in 1893 over rising expenditures for oxygen, they asked the visiting staff to restrict its use.[27] Steadily rising expenses prompted the trustees to order expenditures for 1896 kept within 1891 levels. Trying to reduce costs at the Boston City Hospital, the trustees in 1900 asked the medical staff to use fewer dressings.[28]

Hospital financial needs outstripped the ability of the traditional donor class to meet them. And since American general hospitals are largely voluntary institutions, government support remained minimal in the key early twentieth-century period. That left the patients. Patients had always been required to pay hospital board, as opposed to professional fees, if they could. In hospital after hospital one finds conscious policy decisions to tap the patient resource. Elite eastern institutions, like the Massachusetts General, modified their policies of prohibiting staff physicians from charging professional fees of hospital patients. The purpose of this change in practice was to encourage attending practitioners to bring their private patients to the hospital without fear of losing their fees.[29]

Physicians were no longer to serve the hospital in the spirit of charity. Hospital practice would not be restricted only to elite medical men who could give of their time without direct remuneration. Other institutions opened their staffs, so that greater numbers of practitioners could bring their patients into these hospitals. The private patients of a greatly expanded class of hospital physicians provided the money that kept hospitals going.[30] In the United States in 1922 patient receipts provided more than 65 percent of the income of general hospitals. At the Massachusetts General Hospital patients had contributed $12,000 toward operating expenses of $62,800 in 1870. By 1910 they paid $151,000 of $350,300.[31]

In terms of financial support, the organization and reimbursement of medical practice, and the nature of the patient constituency, the transformation of the hospital from charity to modern medical institution was well underway. One consequence of over half a century of interrelated social and medical changes was that the poor and penniless, whom the institution had originally been meant to serve, became a liability.

Notes

1. Morris J. Vogel, "Boston's Hospitals, 1870-1930: A Social History" (Ph.D. diss., University of Chicago, 1974), chap. 1.

2. Guenter B. Risse, Ronald L. Numbers, and Judith Walzer Leavitt, eds., *Medicine Without Doctors: Home Health Care in American History* (New York, 1977); see specifically the essays by John B. Blake and James H. Cassedy.

3. When an ambulance service was established in Boston in 1871, its stated purpose was to take victims of sudden illness or injury "to their homes or to the hospital" (*Boston Medical and Surgical Journal* 85 [1871]: 340).

4. Henry Sigerist, "An Outline of the Development of the Hospital," *Bulletin of the Institute of the History of Medicine* 4 (1936): 573-81.

5. Charles E. Rosenberg, "The Practice of Medicine in New York A Century Ago," *Bulletin of the History of Medicine* 41 (1976): 224-25, 230-33.

6. J. M. Toner, "Statistics of Regular Medical Associations and Hospitals of the United States," *Transactions of the American Medical Association* 24 (1873): 314-33. Toner included more than 50 mental institutions in his total of 178 hospitals.

7. William H. Williams, *America's First Hospital: The Pennsylvania Hospital, 1751-1841* (Wayne, Pa., 1976), p. 145; for an English example, see George Moore, *Esther Waters, A Novel,* (Boston, 1963), chap. 15; original ed. 1894.

8. Massachusetts General Hospital, *57th Annual Report, 1870,* pp. 13-14.

9. Massachusetts General Hospital, "The Report of a [Trustees'] Committee on the Financial Condition of the Massachusetts General Hospital, 16 February 1865," in Countway Library, Boston; Nathaniel I. Bowditch, *A History of the Massachusetts General Hospital* (Boston, 2nd ed., 1872), p. 454.

10. See, for example, Boston City Hospital, *25th Annual Report, 1888,* pp. 33-34.

11. Children's Hospital (Boston), *15th Annual Report, 1883,* p. 9; *Christian Register,* 8 May 1869.

12. See, for example, Massachusetts General Hospital, Trustees' mss. Records, 3 August 1877, in Massachusetts General Hospital Archives, Boston.

13. Walker Gill Wylie, *Hospitals: Their History, Organization, and Construction* (New York, 1877), pp. 60-62; George S. Hale, "Medical Charities," *National Conference of Charities and Corrections, Proceedings* 2 (1875): 52-66.

14. Henry J. Bigelow, "Fees in Hospitals," *Boston Medical and Surgical Journal* 120 (1889): 378.

15. Quoted in *Boston Medical and Surgical Journal* 106 (1882): 137.

16. Henry J. Bigelow, *Medical Education in America* (Cambridge, 1871), pp. 5-6. See also the article by Gerald Markowitz and David Rosner in this volume.

17. Boston Medical Society, "Circular Letter to Superintendents and Trustees of the Various Hospitals of Boston," dated December 1909, in Richard C. Cabot Papers, Harvard University Archives.

18. State Charities Aid Association of New York, Committee on Hospitals, *New Hospitals Needed in Greater New York* (New York, 1908), p. 56; Sidney E. Goldstein, "The Social Function of the Hospital," *Charities and the Commons* 18 (1907): 163.

19. Talcott Parsons and Renée Fox, "Illness, Therapy, and the Modern Urban Family," *Journal of Social Issues* 8, 4 (1952): 31-34.

20. Boston City Hospital, *24th Annual Report, 1887*, p. 13.

21. Edmund D. Pellegrino, "From the Rational to the Radical: The Sociocultural Impact of Modern Therapeutics," paper presented at the conference on "Two Hundred Years of American Medicine," Philadelphia, December 1976.

22. For data on Boston, see Vogel, "Boston's Hospitals," pp. 240-44.

23. Ivan Illich, *Medical Nemisis: The Expropriation of Health* (New York, 1976), chap. 2.

24. Massachusetts General Hospital, *57th Annual Report, 1870*, pp. 12-13; *97th Annual Report, 1910*, pp. 60-61; *107th Annual Report, 1920*, pp. 98-101.

25. Association of Hospital Superintendants, *7th Annual Conference, 1905*, pp. 116-32, 135, 141.

26. Association of Hospital Superintendants, *5th Annual Conference, 1903*, p. 129; *7th Annual Conference, 1905*, p. 187; *9th Annual Conference, 1907*, pp. 189-90.

27. Massachusetts General Hospital, Trustees' mss. Records, 19 May, 2 June 1893.

28. Massachusetts General Hospital, Trustees' mss. Records, 1 March 1895, 17 January, 10 April 1896; Boston City Hospital, Trustees' mss. Records, 3 April 1900.

29. For a discussion of the Phillips House, a private wing opened at the Massachusetts General Hospital in 1917, see Vogel, "Boston's Hospitals," pp. 217-39.

30. See David Rosner, "A Once Charitable Enterprise: Health Care in Brooklyn, 1890-1915" (Ph.D. diss., Harvard University, 1978) for a fuller account.

31. Massachusetts General Hospital, *57th Annual Report, 1870*, pp. 12-14; *97th Annual Report, 1910*, pp. 60-61.

DAVID ROSNER

7 Business at the Bedside: Health Care in Brooklyn, 1890-1915

Most of us recognize that patients are assigned space in the hospital in accordance with special medical needs. But it is also true that patients are assigned beds according to ability to pay, insurance coverage, and source of referral. Private and semiprivate rooms and small wards are as much a characteristic of contemporary hospitals as are the medical, surgical, and specialty services.[1]

The separation of patients according to economic class and other social factors has a long history. In nineteenth-century America, for instance, wealthier clients generally received care at home or in private doctors' offices; working-class and indigent patients often received care through the out-patient department of hospitals, local dispensaries, workers' associations (lodges), or the charity hospital. While distinctions in service for the rich and the poor have always existed in the American health system as a whole, the incorporation of differing services within the hospital is a relatively recent phenomenon.

Before the turn of the century most non-municipal institutions were charitable in nature and served a primarily working-class population. In that sense, the nineteenth-century hospital was a "one-class" facility. While separate institutions existed for women, blacks, and distinct immigrant groups, internally they were organized in a relatively uniform way. Patients were

I would like to thank Betsy Blackmar, Kathy Conway, Gerald Markowitz, Susan Reverby, and Barbara Rosenkrantz for their helpful comments on drafts of this paper. I would like to acknowledge support from Grant HS 02345, National Center for Health Services Research, HEW, and from the Josiah Macy Foundation.

117

housed in wards with few distinctions based upon the patient's ability to pay.[2] Services were provided at the expense of philanthropists and hospital trustees. As Morris Vogel has illustrated, the nineteenth-century facility served primarily social, rather than medical needs for working class and/or destitute persons.[3]

By the early 1900s a change occurred in the organization of hospital services in charity institutions. During that period the more modern voluntary hospital system arose. This development entailed a dramatic reorganization of the physical space and administrative hierarchy of the hospital. First, the development of class-specific services was a prominent feature of the physical restructuring of the facilities. As trustees sought private patients and their fees, private and semi-private rooms and wards began to displace public and charity wards. Second, as trustees sought to make their institutions more amenable to paying patients, private physicians were admitted to the institutions in the hope that they would bring their patients with them. Ironically, the authority of lay trustees declined as physicians began to exert greater control over the day-to-day services provided their private patients. Third, the care of the charity patient, originally the function of these facilities, was increasingly seen as an inconvenience. In New York the municipal and later the state governments were called upon to bear a larger portion of the financial responsibilities for poor patients in voluntary institutions. This chapter will examine some of the economic pressures that forced trustees in Brooklyn's Progressive Era hospitals to abandon their older, traditional functions as stewards to the poor and to allow their facilities to undergo profound, and at times disruptive, change.

The decline in the charity functions of philanthropic institutions resulted in part from the severe economic crisis that affected many facilities in the wake of the depression of the 1890s. This depression hit Brooklyn's institutions during a period when costs for health care were rapidly rising. In general, institutions in need of money turned to the paying patient as the most likely source. The provision of hospital care ceased to be an act of charity and became a commodity to be bought and sold by those who could afford it.

The move away from charity to pay services was rationalized as part of the larger Progressive Era movements toward order, efficiency, and bureaucracy. However, the hospitals of the period also exemplify changes that do not fit neatly into any historiographic package. The application of business principles to charity hospitals had a different result: other reform movements led to greater emphasis on corporate responsibility, while changes in hospital finance placed the burden on individuals.

I

In the early years of the twentieth century a prominent Brooklyn businessman, Abraham Abraham, became deeply involved in the formation of the Jewish Hospital of Brooklyn. This hospital, Abraham stated, would avoid some of the chronic problems that plagued many of the city's charitable institutions; it would be so organized that it would "not run in debt." Abraham, owner of Abraham and Straus, the city's largest department store, noted that a hospital was not very different from other large enterprises. He believed that "charitable institutions, however laudable and worthy, should be conducted on sound business principles."[4]

Abraham's concern for the development of "business principles" in charity institutions was spurred by a mounting crisis in hospital financing. During the depression years of the 1890s, many of Brooklyn's charity institutions had found their costs rising at the very time that their incomes from philanthropy were shrinking. As economic conditions worsened, working-class patients increasingly demanded hospital service. Ever larger numbers of patients found themselves in need of the traditional services that hospitals provided—shelter and food.[5] As demand increased, so too did the costs of running the facilities. At Brooklyn Hospital, for instance, hospital utilization nearly doubled during the depression years, growing from just over 1,200 patients in 1895 to nearly 2,300 by 1899.[6] At Brooklyn Maternity Hospital the secretary noted a similar dramatic increase. When the necessity for relief [is great], the greater will the demand be upon all charitable institutions for that relief."[7] Others noted that the "times have been hard . . . but it is hard to turn away appeals for aid [from patients]."[8] Even in relatively good times, the use of the hospital by those who needed non-medical services and aid was common. "The coming of Spring always brings remarkable recoveries to some of our most stubborn cases," sarcastically noted one hospital surgeon.[9]

At the very time that patient demand was rising, hospital trustees were faced with another challenge to the financial security of their institutions: costs for medical supplies were growing. As bacteriological practices began to be felt in terms of higher standards of general cleanliness, sterile surroundings, and aseptic surgery, a slow growth in costs for medical supplies and maintenance resulted.[10] During the period, for instance, the use of rubber gloves, sterile bandages, supplies, and equipment became a standard part of hospital expense. At Brooklyn Hospital the average cost for a day of care rose from $.89 in 1890 to $2.78 by 1915.[11]

These two factors, rising patient demand and increasing costs for medical supplies, had a significant impact upon many hospitals. But the ultimate crisis in finance was a result of the fact that philanthropists could no longer make donations large enough to rescue the hospitals from their plight. In the earlier years of the nineteenth century philanthropists could be counted on to cover deficits that were chronic features in most nineteenth-century charity facilities. Many hospitals, in fact, used small but manageable deficits as part of their appeals for funds. A deficit was seen as an indication of the worth of the institution, just as modest want was seen as proof of the worthiness of one of the hospital's inmates. Philanthropists were more willing to give to an institution that had a small end-of-the-year deficit.

The depression forced philanthropists to reasses this long-standing practice. Hospital deficits were now growing larger every year. Furthermore, the trustees and philanthropists themselves were feeling the pinch of this long and severe depression. They were less willing and able to part with their money than they had been in the past.

In sum, charity was proving an inadequate means of supporting the hospitals. Trustees and managers alike remarked that there was a "tendency of charitable bequests to diminish" and that this was "a matter of great concern."[12] One trustee noted that when the "financial depression struck this land, we were obliged to struggle on as best as we could." The president of Brooklyn Hospital reported in 1895 that the hospital's financial condition was poor. "On the financial side," he remarked, "we have not been able to meet our expenses."[13] The president of one of Brooklyn's oldest specialty facilities summed up the crisis that plagued many institutions during the depression years: "Not only are the demands upon the hospital greater and the expenses consistently increasing, but the sources of revenue from individual subscription are diminishing."[14]

The economic crunch that hit Brooklyn's hospitals served as a warning to the trustees of some institutions and as a death blow to others. During the 1890s, for instance, no fewer than five of Brooklyn's largest hospitals closed their doors. One trustee noted that Memorial Hospital "had an uphill and hopeless struggle. . . . Disaster after disaster overtook them until burdened with debt, [it] . . . had to succumb."[15] When the Williamsburg Hospital in a large working—class neighborhood closed in the early 1900s, the trustees were deeply in debt and could not gather the necessary funds. Homeopathic Hospital struggled through the depression and was taken over by the city, $70,000 in debt.[16] By 1899 one of the prominent hospitals reported that it owed $27,000 to various banks and that a substantial portion of its endowment had been spent.[17]

By the early years of the twentieth century, the general crisis in hospital finance had become so widely recognized that a "Conference on Hospital Needs and Hospital Finances" was called for by administrators and the Charity Organization Society. In the announcement for the meeting the sponsors noted that "heavy annual deficits are the rule rather than the exception" in most of the city's hospitals.[18]

In New York and Brooklyn alike, trustees and superintendents recognized that the charity system was breaking down. A few wealthy benefactors and local annual subscription drives were an inadequate means of financing the city's private institutions.[19] Hospital administrators and trustees were faced with the necessity of finding alternative sources of financial support. As Mr. Abraham pointed out in his own inimicable way, "In reading over the reports of [Brooklyn's] charitable [institutions] they all ring . . . the one 'leit motif' and the one refrain: appeal upon appeal to the public to help pay off large mortgages and other indebtedness."[20] A new means of financing charitable institutions was clearly needed. During the early 1900s, in the wake of a severe depression, trustees in many facilities began to look toward pay patients as a new source of income and as a means of forestalling the collapse of their facilities.

II

The traditional financial bases of most Brooklyn hospitals had been the benevolence of wealthy trustees, patrons, church-goers, and other private individuals. They participated in hospital work for many reasons: partly from a sense of noblesse oblige, in order to gain or maintain recognition as community leaders, or because of their interest in social control and cultural hegemony. The objects of their benevolence had uniformly been the poor and working class of the city.

But by the early 1900s it was clear that there were good economic reasons for reluctant trustees to abandon their uniform objective of servicing the poor.[21] Scientific medicine was changing the character of the old charity facilities, wealthier patients seemed ready to utilize the hospital, and poorer persons were a severe drain on the resources of many facilities. Hospital income could be increased significantly if, first, patients could be convinced to pay for their care and, second, if a greater number of wealthier clients could be attracted to the facility. Most trustees still maintained that charity was the proper justification for the hospital. But, increasingly, "free" or "charity" patients were seen as a growing burden to financially pressed trustees.[22]

Some trustees felt that the number of poor persons admitted should be limited, while others felt that more extreme measures were necessary. Some actually refused care to those who could not pay. Especially during the depression, trustees learned that limiting the number of working-class patients who needed "free" care was the only means open to them to cut costs. "Early last winter, it became apparent that something must be done to procure immediate pecuniary relief," one hospital president remarked. "A cruel fact stared us in the face. . . . We had been rolling up a debt. . . . After careful study, our advisors decided that . . . we should limit the number of inmates."[23] At a small Williamsburg facility, trustees reluctantly observed that there was a "limit to our resources."[24]

During bad times it was clear that no facility could not ac-
comodate everyone. But this practice of excluding poorer patients was carried on past the immediate depression years and
became an axiom of hospital administration during the early
twentieth century. At the Brooklyn Hospital, for instance, the
trustees began to see the paying patient as an important source
of income and the free patient as an increasingly expendable
burden. "Further space in the wards must be prepared for the
[pay] service if we wish to further increase our income from
this source," the vice-president of the board of trustees declared
in 1899.[25] By 1902 the trustee "decided to shut out part of the
charity patients [in order to] keep expenditures down." The
hospital, the president remarked, had previously "attempted to
do more charity work than it could afford."[26] In 1892 only 12
percent of this hospital's income came directly from the patient.
By 1905 nearly 45 percent was derived from patient payments.[27]

Although changes in hospital organization and administration
had begun earlier in the nineteenth century, the depression of
the 1890s greatly accelerated them. Specifically, the deficits
made the businessman's cry for efficiency, bureaucracy, and
business practices more convincing to hospital boards. The
deficits also undermined the charity orientation of many
trustees. Furthermore, the crisis led to the hospitals' new
dependence on physicians who claimed they could supply them
with a new class of patients who could *pay* for care. This meant
that new amenities and services would have to be provided in
order to attract doctors and their patients. Advanced technology
services that were of interest to practitioners were introduced.
Private rooms, wards, doctoring, and nursing had to be provided
for wealthier clients. In quick succession hospital boards voted
to expand their visiting and attending staffs. Brooklyn Hospital
increased the number of associated physicians from fewer than
a dozen in 1890 to nearly sixty by 1915. At Methodist the
number rose from about fifteen to fifty-five during the same
period.[28]

The introduction of private physicians into the charity hospital had a profound and long-lasting effect on the organization of
these facilities. First, trustees had traditionally seen the hospital
as their private responsibility and the arrival of large numbers of

physicians meant a new challenge to their authority as benefactors and stewards to the poor. Second, the physicians had a substantial impact on the underlying purpose of these institutions.
Hospitals became more clearly defined as places for medical
treatment rather than shelters for the poor and homeless.

While doctors changed the tone of the wards, businessmen on
the boards changed the tenor of board meetings. Like Abraham
Abraham at the Jewish Hospital, businessmen gained a new importance at other institutions as well. The president of the
board at the small Bushwick Hospital announced that H. C.
Bohack, who had recently opened a chain of food stores, had
joined the board. As the president saw it, "the business interests
of the hospital could not more effectively be safeguarded" than
by directly involving such men. At Brooklyn Hospital, Charles
Pratt became president of the board. Pratt, whose family had
founded the oil refineries in Greenpoint and who managed John
D. Rockefeller's East Coast refineries, made substantial changes
at this institution as well.[29]

The direct effects of the involvement of all of these individuals
was ambiguous. But they certainly did bring a business point of
view to challenge the norms of the hospital boards. Managers
and trustees, who ascribed to older paternalist ideologies, found
themselves hard put to defend their roles as financial stewards
when they themselves had no solution to the chronic financial
crises. Older ideals began to be played down and newer business
ones placed in their stead. Some trustees were often put in a
quandary, denying that the facility had changed into a business.
The president of one hospital cried out that his facility was "a
work of mercy . . . not a business."[30] Another declared in 1907
that "we are not in hospital work to make money."[31]

At the end of the Progressive Era one prominent surgeon
commented on a paper about a Brooklyn hospital published in
the *Bulletin of the Taylor Society,* the society dedicated to
scientific management. The paper sought to apply principles of
scientific management to the organization of the hospital. In
commenting on the paper, Ernest Codman, a Boston surgeon
concerned with the rationalization of the hospital, observed
that "charitable hospitals have become businesses and are . . .
wolves in sheep's clothing."[32] Clearly the older charitable impetus for hospital work was waning as the financial crunch hit

many facilities. Charity clients were a burden. As one trustee pointed out, "Additional income must be had, and that can come only from pay patients."[33]

III

The turn away from charity affected the working-class patients in two ways. First, trustees sometimes converted "free" wards into pay wards or rooms. This took away space previously available for indigent patients. Second, trustees more often began to charge working-class patients for services that were previously provided free. Different levels of services were devised for those willing to pay. Also, existing ethnic and other social distinctions functioned to convince those who would afford it not to use a "lower grade" of service. This divided different working-class groups into separate quarters and perpetuated existing divisions within this class. Moreover, the poorest of the patients, those unable to pay anything for their care, were increasingly seen as the *source* of the financial problems of the hospital rather than the *victims* of the crisis in hospital finance. The "fruitful cause for the annual deficiency in the hospitals," remarked one hospital manager in New York, "is the large number of free patients." If the former objects of charity did not pay for their care, then they were now defined as the problem. "If hospital patients had more honor and pride, I do not think there would be any large deficiency," he concluded.[34] Instead of seeing the poorer patients as needy and consequently deserving of care, hospital administrators viewed neediness as a moral failing of the patient.

If hospitals now charged only wealthier clients for their care while maintaining services to working-class patients, the practical effect of this reorientation toward the paying patient might not have been terribly important. This was not the case, however. In Brooklyn there was no ready and willing group of middle-class patients eager to use charity facilities long associated with the most degrading type of care; only special services and new accomodations could attract the middle class. The small, financially unstable facilities of Brooklyn could hardly afford to build additional wings and services. Consequently, space for free patients was often converted into space for pay patients and, more often than not, formerly charity patients were required to pay for their care. At Brooklyn Hospital, for instance, the number of "free" patients grew from about 1,000 to 1,600 during the depression years and immediately following but then dropped dramatically from 1,600 in 1900 to 1,200 in 1903. As noted earlier, it was 1900 when the hospital trustees announced that beds in the charity ward would be converted into pay beds in order to increase income. At the same point the number of paying patients began to grow dramatically, rising from just over 200 in 1899 to 1,400 by 1911. The number of private room patients, never a large number in any particular year, remained relatively small throughout the period. In 1895, 16.3 percent of all patient days were used for pay-ward patients. By 1905 this category had grown to 44.5 percent.[35]

While the change in hospital space usage was dramatic, the change in the class of the hospital patient was not. This leads to the conclusion that the pay wards were primarily filled by the same class of patients that previously used the free hospital space. In Brooklyn Hospital, for example, white-collar workers accounted for 13 percent of the patients in 1892 and grew slowly to 21 percent by 1902. The bulk of the patients were still working class—only now they had to pay for their care. On the one hand, it was "obvious that there can be no very great increase in income from [pay patients] unless the accommodations . . . are increased at the expense of space alloted now to those [who] . . . cannot pay at all."[36] On the other hand, charging the same group of patients who had previously used the facility for free accomplished much the same thing. At Brooklyn Hospital this appeared to be what was done. The trustees periodically transformed charity wards into pay wards when income was needed.[37]

The internal organization of many facilities was also greatly affected by the change from charity to pay. Hospitals throughout Brooklyn began to assign bed space to patients according to social and economic criteria rather than medical need. Within the context of the growing acceptance of patient payment as a legitimate source of hospital revenue, it became mandatory for hospital managers to make services distinctly different for the charity and paying patients in order to convince patients that, if they could afford to, they should use the paying service. The source of referral, whether the social service and business office or the private practitioner, gave some basis for differentiating between those able to pay and those who were indigent. But the offering of different services provided a surer means of selecting out patients. The right to a private physician, smaller wards or private rooms, and better food were immediately seen as prerogatives of the pay service. In contrast, charity patients were provided with care that was determined by the administration rather than by a private physician. Private patients were serviced in entirely different quarters. Some called for separate facilities for the rich and the poor. *The Journal of the American Medical Association* pointed out that the "absolute segregation of charity patients from pay patients" was necessary if the wealthier patient was to be convinced to pay for his or her care. "Those who really have no means will perforce go to the genuine charity hospitals, while few of those who have any income will sink their pride so far as to enter an institution patronized by none but the destitute. . . . When the only alternative is a pay hospital where none are treated free, the deed is done. So long as rich and poor are treated under one roof, the well-to-do will not scrupple at getting free treatment [since] no stigma attaches to residence in an institution where many pay their way." Separation of services along class lines was necessary to guarantee that clients would, if able, pay for their treatment.[38]

The transformation of the structure and organization of the hospital preceded the introduction of wealthier clients. In many facilities private rooms and pay wards remained empty until after World War I. But in the interim many working-class patients were refused entrance, charged for services previously provided free, and made to feel that the hospital was no longer concerned with their well-being. Some poorer patients were able to scrape together the necessary cash and enter the new "pay" wards. Others were forced to seek care in the growing system of public institutions. Still others were taken into the voluntary institutions only when payment from the city coffers was guaranteed.

The relationship between the charity hospitals and the city government had a long history, dating back to the 1840s. At that time the city of Brooklyn issued lump-sum payments to charity facilities so that these institutions would care for poor persons who were deemed to be proper recipients of the city's protection. But in the early 1900s this flat-grant system of payments was transformed into per capita, per diem payment schemes based upon a means test of all patients. The means test and new grant system further accelerated the administrators' plan to exclude those whose expenses were not covered.[39]

It would be naive to conclude that trustees consciously reorganized hospital services along social class lines. Rather, such actions to develop class-distinct services were an outgrowth of a complex process of financial, intellectual, and social changes that had little to do with the trustees and superintendents themselves. Once patients were accepted as a reasonable source of income, the selling of health services—through private rooms, wards, private nursing, doctors, and special amenities—swiftly arose. Most trustees, in fact, had little or no understanding of how profoundly their institutions would change once patients were turned to as a source of income. In fact, the trustees' own declining authority was further threatened by the very practitioners whom they needed to save the hospital. These practitioners brought with them a growing expertise and professional authority that would quickly allow them to bypass the trustee in influence.[40] The decisions of trustees to change the base of their financial support had a deleterious effect on their own position as well.

By the end of the Progressive Era the modern outlines of an internally fragmented hospital system were apparent in many of Brooklyn's facilities. Not only were physicians much more prominent, and not only were their interests reflected in an increasingly complex medical organization, but the hospital itself was now split between public and private services. In 1916 the Brooklyn Hospital distributed a brochure with an illustration of the hospital on its cover. Engraved across the roof of one of the two wings of the hospital was the word *"PUBLIC."* Across the roof of the other was the word *"PRIVATE."* Between these stood the administration building that kept two worlds of medicine far apart.[41]

Notes

1. See, for example, the voluminous literature on the organization of ward, room, and private service within hospitals. The most widely known critique of such service differentiations comes from various Health PAC publications. For instance, see Health PAC's *The American Health Empire* (New York: Random House, 1970), and David Kotelchuck, ed. *Prognosis Negative: Crisis in the Health Care System* (New York: Vintage Books, 1976).

2. Morris Vogel, "Patrons, Practitioners, and Patients: The Voluntary Hospital in Mid-Victorian Boston," in *Victorian America,* ed. by Daniel W. Howe (Philadelphia: University of Pennsylvania Press, 1976), pp. 120-21: "Patients who could not, and in most cases were forbidden to, pay any fee." Other authors have also noted the organization of charity hospitals in the nineteenth century; see, for example, Charles Rosenberg, "And Heal The Sick: The Hospital and Patient in 19th Century America," *Journal of Social History* 10 (June 1977): 482-97.

3. See, in addition to the above mentioned article, Morris Vogel, "Boston's Hospitals: 1880-1930" (Ph.D. Diss., University of Chicago, 1974); also Susan Reverby's article in this volume and her thesis in progress, American Studies Program, Boston University.

4. Jewish Hospital of Brooklyn, *2nd Annual Report,* 1903, p. 10.

5. Such social (i.e., non-medical) functions were an important aspect of nineteenth-century hospital care. See note 3, above, for a more extended discussion of the nineteenth-century facility.

6. See Brooklyn Hospital, *Annual Reports,* 1895, 1899.

7. Brooklyn Maternity Hospital, *Annual Report,* 1896, p. 11.

8. See Brooklyn Nursery and Infants Hospital, *Annual Report,* 1896, p. 15; and Methodist Hospital, *Annual Report,* 1896, p. 15, for similar comments.

9. "Men and Women Who Feign Disease: Hospitals . . . Have To Be Constantly On Guard Against Malingerers," *New York Tribune,* 1 May 1904, sec. 2, p. 2.

10. An analysis of costs at a number of Brooklyn facilities indicates that general housekeeping, maintenance, and other costs grew along with a slow rise in the category of "medical supplies." But patient demand was of great significance as well.

11. The statistical information in this article is drawn from the annual reports of the various institutions; see, for example, Brooklyn Hospital, *Annual Reports,* 1890-1915, for the above quoted material.

12. Frederick Sturges, "What Managers of Hospitals Say About Their Financial Problems," *Charities* 12 (January 1904): 32.

13. See, for example, Memorial Hospital, *10th Annual Report,* 1898, p. 16; Brooklyn Eye and Ear Hospital, *13th Annual Report,* 1898. In 1896 the directors noted that the "sources of revenue . . . are diminishing" (Brooklyn Hospital, *Annual Report,* 1895, p. 6). See also, Charity Organization Society of New York, *Report,* 1900: "Several of the large private hospitals are having increased difficulty in securing . . . funds [from philanthropists]."

14. Brooklyn Eye and Ear Hospital, *29th Annual Report,* 1896; Methodist Hospital, *Annual Report,* 1894, p. 19; and other numerous contemporary statements.

15. Jewish Hospital of Brooklyn, *2nd Annual Report,* 1903, p. 8. Also Memorial Hospital's *Annual Reports* for the previous ten years, which outline its financial collapse.

16. Jewish Hospital, *2nd Annual Report,* 1903, p. 8. See also "Williamsburg Hospital Closes," *New York Tribune,* 16 January 1903, p. 7: "The trustees could see no way . . . they could obtain the necessary money to continue [and] they decided to abandon the work before going further

into debt." See "City Takes The Hospital," *B. D. Eagle,* 26 July 1900 (The Homeopathic Hospital became Cumberland Hospital); "Homeopathic Hospital to Close This Evening," *B. D. Eagle,* 31 March 1900; "Hospital Bill Hearing To-Day," *B. D. Eagle,* 7 March 1900; "Anent the Homeopaths," *B. D. Eagle,* 6 March 1900.

17. Editorial, *The Trained Nurse and Hospital Review,* 29 (September 1902): 194. See also Brooklyn Hospital, *Annual Report,* 1899, p. 8: "Deficits of recent years [have] resulted in a floating debt of about twenty-seven thousand dollars."

18. "A Hospital Conference in New York," *Charities,* 11 March 1905, p. 565.

19. Frederick Sturges, "What The Managers Of The Hospitals . . . Say About Their Financial Problems," *Charities* 12 (January 1904): 32. Sturges continues saying that "the founders and the charter members of the great private hospitals, and their direct descendants are the ones who are now principally carrying them, and it is extraordinarily difficult to interest the younger generation. . . ."

20. Jewish Hospital, *2nd Annual Report,* 1903, p. 10. See also Frank Tucker, "The Public Conscience and the Hospital," *Charities* 13 (December 1904): 285; and Tucker, "Hospital Situation in New York," *Charities* 12 (January 1904): 31.

21. Morris Vogel has outlined some of the demographic factors such as changes in housing patterns and in the make-up of the work force. He has also noted some internal reasons for the introduction of private patients. See notes 2 and 3, above.

22. Jewish Hospital, *Annual Report,* 1903, p. 11.

23. Nursery and Infants Hospital, 23rd *Annual Report,* p. 16. See also, Memorial Hospital for Women and Children, *Annual Report,* 1898, p. 18.

24. Brooklyn Eastern District Dispensary and Hospital, *Annual Report,* 1891, p. 8.

25. Brooklyn Hospital, *Annual Report,* 1899, p. 8, and Brooklyn Hospital, *Annual Report,* 1900, p. 7.

26. Editorial Comment, *The Trained Nurse and Hospital Review,* 29 (September 1902): 194. I would like to thank Susan Reverby for providing this citation.

27. This tendency to depend increasingly upon patient payments is general to most of Brooklyn's hospitals. See, for example the annual reports of Methodist, Jewish, and other institutions.

28. See medical directories and medical registers of New York, Brooklyn and New Jersey for these years. These publications put out by the local medical societies contain lists of physicians and their affiliations for specific years.

29. Bushwick and Bushwick Central Hospital, *11th Annual Report,* March 1904-1905, p. 10. See also Obituary, "H. C. Bohack," *New York Times,* 18 September 1931, p. 23: "President of Bohack Chain of 746 stores . . . H. C. Bohack was born in Germany in 1865, opened his first store in 1885. Had five stores by 1900, president of a realty corporation, director of People's National Bank, Guarantee Title and Mortgage Co., Brooklyn National Life Insurance Co., Williamsburg Savings Bank, Manhat-

tan Trust." See also Brooklyn Hospital, *Minutes,* 1912-1914, for detailed description of the numerous changes that Pratt made in hospital organization.

30. Lutheran Hospital Association, *Annual Report,* 1914, p. 2. See also Brooklyn Homeopathic Maternity, *Annual Report,* 1899, p. 12, in which the secretary disdainfully notes that "other maternities in this and our sister city . . . demand pay for every patient [while] we work largely for charity."

31. Bushwick Hospital, *Annual Report,* 1906-1907, p. 15.

32. See Robert L. Dickinson, "Hospital Organization As Shown By Charts of Personnel and Power Functions," *Bulletin of the Taylor Society,* 3 (October 1917), pp. 1-11, and Codman's response.

33. Lutheran Hospital Association, *Annual Report,* 1914, p. 21; Methodist Hospital, *Annual Report,* 1894, p. 20. See also Long Island College Hospital, *Hospital Yearbook,* 1919, p. 35, for a later statement of the increasing pressure to get paying patients into the hospital. A. C. Bunn, "Church Hospitals," *Brooklyn Medical Journal* 15 (September 1909): 508.

34. Ogden Chisholm, "Financial Problems of New York's Hospitals," *Charities,* 12 (2 June 1904): 38.

35. See the annual reports of Brooklyn Hospital for 1890-1915; also Charles Rosenberg, "The Shaping of the American Hospital 1880-1914," unpublished manuscript, 1978, for confirmation that many hospitals found their private services empty during the period.

36. Frank Tucker, "The Hospital Situation in New York," *Charities* 12 (January 1904): 30; A. C. Bunn, "Church Hospitals," *Brooklyn Medical Journal* 15 (September 1901): 510. See also Charlotte Aikens, "Relation of the Training School to the Hospital Deficit Problem," *The Trained Nurse* 37 (September 1910): 157: "The Extension and Improvement of the Pay Patient Department . . . is one of the remedies for deficits that is meeting with general favor."

37. Brooklyn Hospital, *Executive Minutes* 5 (23 January 1901): 104: "Resolved that the private accomodations of the Hospital be increased by converting Wards 10, 11, 12, and 13 or so much thereof as may be necessary, into Pay Wards without material alterations or expense. . . ."

38. Editorial, "Abolish The Hospital Grafter", *Journal of the American Medical Association* 44 (27 May 1905): 1691.

39. For a fuller description of the city's involvement, see David Rosner, "A Once Charitable Enterprise: Health Care in Brooklyn, 1890-1915" (Ph.D. diss., History of Science Department, Harvard University, 1978), chap. 3.

40. See Gerald E. Markowitz and David K. Rosner, "Doctors in Crisis: Medical Education and Medical Reform During The Progressive Era, 1895-1915." in this volume for an expanded discussion of the rising professional status of the physician.

41. See brochure and illustration that is reproduced in "Brooklyn's Oldest Hospital Built Anew," *The Modern Hospital* 7 (November 1916): 361-66.

8   *He Who Pays the Piper:*
Foundations, the Medical
Profession, and
Medical Education

Many historical forces have shaped contemporary medical practice and medical education. These range from the specific reform strategies of the profession's leadership to material and ideological support from dominant industrial and corporate capitalist classes. Recent critical analysis has focused on the profession's role in promoting its own interests and on medicine as an institution of social control—both perceptions long obscured by the sacred robes in which medicine has been clothed.[1] Little empirical attention, however, has been paid to the roles of dominant classes and their powerful institutional instruments in molding modern American medicine.[2] This chapter examines how the Rockefeller foundations used their immense wealth to force specific reforms in medical education, reforms the philanthropies' chief architect believed would make medicine serve the needs of capitalist society rather than the interests of the medical profession.[3]

Foundations, and chiefly the Rockefeller philanthropies, financed the most important reforms in medical education. From 1910 to the 1930s foundations gave some $300 million for medical education and research, earning Rosemary Stevens' designation as "the most vital outside force in effecting changes in medical education after 1910."[4] As the suppliers of needed capital, they were often able to dictate terms to the profession.

As Diana Long Hall has argued, the relationship between foundations and the medical profession often was one of "mutual seduction."[5] The medical profession was no innocent being led astray, nor were the foundations totally hegemonic in defining how this affair would proceed. Similarly, neither the medical profession nor the foundations presented monolithic viewpoints. In fact, the divisions within each group were a key to the marriage of convenience.

The Flexner Report

One of the crucial dates in this romance was 1910, the year the Carnegie Foundation published Abraham Flexner's merciless attack on contemporary medical education. Flexner flailed most medical schools for their failure to enforce preliminary education requirements for applicants, their inadequate facilities and training in both laboratory sciences and clinical medicine, and their overproduction of doctors. He pinned much of the responsibility for these problems on "commercial" medical schools—proprietary schools set up and run by physicians. For Flexner, the scientific model of the Johns Hopkins medical school embodied all that was good and proper in medical education.[6]

These criticisms and the recommendations that followed from them—putting medical schools under the control of universities, raising and enforcing the preliminary education requirements, lengthening and improving the curriculum and facilities, and cutting the number of schools and their output of doctors—had all been part of the profession's own decades-old strategy to upgrade their status and incomes as well as their technical skills. The profession's main vehicles for implementing this strategy were the American Medical Association, its Council on Medical Education, the Association of American Medical Colleges, and state medical licensing boards.

Flexner's report aided a process that was already underway. The rate of consolidation and elimination of medical schools was as rapid before the report as after. Between 1904 and 1915 some ninety-two schools closed their doors or merged, forty-four of them in the first six years to 1909 and forty-eight in the second six years to 1915.[7]

The report's direct impact on the profession was moderate, but its consequences were indirectly monumental. As Flexner himself pointed out, the report spoke to the public on behalf of the medical reform movement. It helped "educate" the public to accept scientific medicine, and most important, it "educated" wealthy men and women to channel their philanthropy to support research-oriented scientific medical education. The Flexner report and the Carnegie Foundation's support brought economic and political power into the war as partisans of the "regular" doctors *cum* scientific medical men.

Within a year following the report's publication, the General Education Board (GEB), the first Rockefeller Foundation created in 1902, entered the fray in earnest. By 1920 the GEB had appropriated nearly $15 million for medical education and by 1929 a total of more than $78 million.[8] The matching grant policy, requiring the recipient institution to raise an equal sum itself, greatly increased the impact of their funds. Because the foundation grants were conditional on specific reforms in the medical schools, the foundations exerted a major influence. They forced schools to adopt a research orientation, required teaching hospitals to subordinate their autonomy and patient care to the needs and authority of a university medical school, and established salaried clinical professorships.

The Carnegie Foundation provided its resources to the leading medical professionals. The Flexner report united the interests of elite practitioners, scientific medical faculty, and the wealthy capitalist class. The report validated the elite professionals and enabled them to speak to philanthropists with a single voice, amplified by the Carnegie Foundation. The General Education Board, however, interjected a discordant note into this harmonious relationship.

The General Education Board: Medical Education Reform Gets a Different Drummer

In the spring of 1911 Frederick T. Gates, John D. Rockefeller's chief lieutenant for his financial empire and the architect of Rockefeller medical and other philanthropies, invited Abraham Flexner to lunch. As Flexner years later recalled the momentous meeting, Gates complimented him on Bulletin Number Four and asked him: "What would you do if you had a million dollars with which to make a start in reorganizing medical education in the United States?"

"Without a moment's hesitation," Flexner recommended giving it all to Dr. William Welch and the Johns Hopkins Medical School. Flexner could not have recommended anyone in medicine more dear to Gates, who then asked Flexner to obtain a leave from the Carnegie Foundation for a few weeks to go to Baltimore as an agent of the General Education Board and report back on his findings at Johns Hopkins. Flexner was delighted and went off to Baltimore assured that the million dollars was available.[9]

In Baltimore Flexner went directly to Welch and explained that the GEB might add a million dollars to the Johns Hopkins Medical School endowment, and that he was there to study the situation and report back to Gates. Welch arranged a dinner that night at the Maryland Club and invited two of Hopkins' most illustrious medical faculty, Franklin P. Mall, an anatomist who in effect represented the medical science faculty, and William S. Halsted, a surgeon and de facto representative of the clinical faculty.

Mall spoke without hesitation: "If the school could get a sum of approximately $1 million, in my judgment there is only one thing that we ought to do with it—use every penny of its income for the purpose of placing upon a salary basis the heads and assistants in the leading *clinical* departments." That, Mall added, "is the great reform which needs now to be carried through."[10]

Mall's suggestion was the focus of Flexner's report to Gates. Flexner recommended a grant of $1.5 million to reorganize the medical, surgical, obstetrical, and pediatric departments, placing the clinical faculty on a full-time basis. The "full-time plan" would require the clinical faculty, at that time earning roughly $20,000 to $35,000 a year from consultations, to become salaried employees of the medical school and to *turn over all their consultation fees to the school.* Incomes would thus drop to $10,000 for a department head, still a very high salary for the period, and $2,500 for his assistants.

Flexner's report greatly impressed Gates. The recommendations was informally adopted as policy, and, at Gates' request,

Flexner returned to Baltimore, personally explained it to Welch, and gave him an informal and confidential assurance that a Hopkins application for $1.5 million to institute the reforms would be approved by the GEB. It would be up to Welch to convince his faculty and the university trustees to make the reform, for it was to be the only basis of the GEB's grant. "No pressure was used," Flexner recalled, "no inducement was held out." Just $1.5 million.[11]

When Flexner brought the proposal to the GEB, the full-time plan already had a powerful advocate within the Board. Three years earlier Gates had been instrumental in establishing the strict full-time provision for physician-researchers at the Rockefeller Institute's new hospital.[12] Gates believed the full-time plan would encourage the application of science to medicine and reduce the independence of the medical profession.

Gates—a director of industry, finance, and philanthropy—believed, as did other men in his position, in the *usefulness* of science and technology. Science would discover the causes of diseases, and technology could develop the means to prevent or cure disease. But medical science could neither relieve the misery of the world nor make the work force healthier if people could not afford its services. The financial independence of the medical profession was an obstacle to bringing the benefits of science to the people. "This practice of fixing his own price granted to American physicians by custom," Gates wrote to the other *GEB* trustees, "is the greatest present American obstruction to the usefulness of the science of medicine. For it confines the benefits of the science too largely to the rich, when it is the rightful inheritance of all the people alike, and the public health requires they have it."[13]

Commercialism was fine in the economic sectors that should be reserved for profit making, but in medicine it violated the needs of capitalist society. The full-time plan was adopted by the GEB as its central policy in medical education to help, as board member Jerome D. Greene put it, "in abating commercialism in the medical profession."[14] If the elite, standard-setting medical schools supported by the GEB adopted the fixed price schedule for medical services, Gates argued, "public sentiment, in no time, will enforce those schedules, if reasonable, not only throughout their cities but other cities and finally the country at large."[15]

136

The full-time plan played a central role in foundation funding of medical education for the following important decade of development. The new arrangement altered the relationship of the medical profession to university medical schools. And at the same time it caused deep divisions between the reform-minded elite practitioners in the medical societies and the Rockefeller philanthropies.

Full Time: "Gold or Glory"

As Flexner himself has pointed out, the full-time plan for clinical faculty was suggested to him by Mall, though it had first been advocated publicly in 1902 by Lewellys F. Barker, a former colleague of Mall's at Baltimore and then a professor of anatomy at Chicago.[16] The earlier origins of the idea can be traced to more obscure beginnings in German medical laboratories, but its introduction to the United States is of interest here.

The full-time plan was first instituted in the United States in 1893 when the Johns Hopkins Medical School opened its doors. Because of the new school's emphasis on research and the widespread experience that local practitioners do little research in the laboratory sciences, the university provided full-time faculty positions in anatomy, physiology, pathology, and pharmacology. The models for the Hopkins reform were the German medical laboratories and universities where Welch and the other Hopkins medical faculty received their scientific training. For some of the new faculty who had previously split their time between private practice and teaching laboratory sciences, the Hopkins plan meant giving up an income of $10,000 a year or more, in return for a salary of $3,000 or $4,000. But the bright young men who were actively recruited were, like Welch and Mall, struggling to survive without private practice.[17]

Mall saw the struggle over the full-time plan as a contest between the clinical faculty and practicing physicians, on the one hand, and the laboratory science faculty, on the other. Reform practitioners had demanded full-time laboratory faculty for the first two years of basic science in medical school, and now "it falls to us to demand of the last two years of medicine what they demanded of the first two." With a sense of victory occasioned by the GEB's proposal to Hopkins, Mall added that "the day of reckoning is at hand." The lesser salaries of full-time faculty should not deter brilliant men and women from entering the field. As Mall liked to put the issue, a physician must choose "which 'G' to worship—Gold or Glory."[18]

Other laboratory science faculty had similar motivations. Many were undoubtedly drawn to the medical sciences partly for the field's growing prestige, partly for their interest in the single-minded pursuit possible in a laboratory, and partly for escape from hustling patients and dealing with the mundane business of medical practice.

To the laboratory scientists, limiting clinicians to their salaries would accomplish several things at once. First, they believed that medicine should be fundamentally a science devoted to finding the biophysical causes of disease and less an art of bedside diagnosis and hopeful therapies. Second, since the medical sciences prospered most with faculty devoting themselves entirely to research and teaching, it followed in their thinking that clinical instruction would also benefit from the clinical faculty's singular devotion to research and teaching. Third, since the medical school competed for time and energy with the clinician's private practice, eliminating private practice would unify and rationalize the organization of the medical school. Clinicians would no longer be responsible to an outside practice. Finally, eliminating clinicians' private practices would unify the *material* interests of all the faculty in the medical school. Clinical faculty, leaving behind large and fashionable private practices, would derive their income and prestige from the same source as the laboratory faculty. Traditionally, American practitioners had used their faculty positions in medical schools to build large, prestigious, and very lucrative private practices. The proposed full-time plan would reduce such practices, making the main clinical faculty captives of the medical school, with loyalties no longer divided between personally lucrative consultations and the needs of the school for research and teaching.

Some practitioners as well as academic doctors were mindful of the need for faculty who would commit themselves mainly to teaching. As early as 1900, the *Journal of the American Medical Association* argued that clinical departments should be headed by men "who are properly paid and of whom more may be demanded than of those who regard their clinical services merely as a means of rapidly acquiring a large private clien-

138

tele."[19] But as news of the Hopkins plan spread, the outrage among private practitioners grew. The AMA appointed a special committee on the reorganization of clinical teaching. Its prestigious chairman, Victor Vaughan of Michigan tried to steer a middle course, rejecting expressing the committee's considerable skepticism of the full-time plan. Vaughan concluded that, even if the plan were ideal, it would not be feasible for any but a few medical schools that were well-endowed.[20]

Many clinical faculty charged that full-time medical school faculty, based in laboratories and wards, made "poor practitioners" because they were more concerned with research than with patients as suffering human beings. They claimed that without a private practice a physician would lose touch with the real practice of medicine and be a poor example for medical students. William Osler, the renowned professor of medicine at Hopkins who had introduced a number of reforms in clinical teaching, had always been an advocate of "medicine as art" as well as science. He frequently argued with Mall, who conceived of medicine as simply a research science. When Osler left Hopkins for Oxford in 1904, he bitterly conceded to Mall: "Now I go, and you have your way."[21] The iniation of the full-time plan at Hopkins must not have surprised him, and he wrote from England his severe criticisms of the proposed change. Similarly, the highly regarded Society of Clinical Surgery, including such celebrated surgeons as Charles Mayo and George Crile, registered their opposition to the plan. Other general and specialty societies joined the chorus.[22]

Practitioner attacks on the full-time plan exposed their ideological, material, and political differences with academic physicians, particularly the laboratory scientists. Although the shared commitment of practitioners and academics to promoting scientific medicine had united them at the end of the nineteenth century, differences quickly developed as to just what that meant. Academics differed with practitioners over the relative weight of science and art in medicine, the financial interests of practitioner-clinicians, and who should control medicine.

Medical scientists and their foundation allies believed that medicine was at its best as an exact science, isolating variables in the laboratory and finding a cure under very precise laboratory conditions. Practitioners, in the business of selling cures to patients, seldom saw the relevance of laboratory controls to treating individuals in the real world. With all their deficiencies the proprietary schools had, in the words of Rosemary Stevens, "at least been firmly attuned to the average practitioner."[23] The medical ideology implicit in the full-time plan was now driving practitioners and academics apart.

Whether the practitioners were driven more by their commitment to practice or by consideration for their bank accounts is, of course, a moot question. The issues were so intertwined that it was never clear whether the argument that medicine is an art was simply a ruse to hide pecuniary motives. Clinicians fiercely defended their material interests against the infringements of the full-time plan. Arthur Dean Bevan, the powerful chairman of the AMA's Council on Medical Education, denounced the plan as "unethical and illegal" for depriving clinical faculty of their fees.[24]

Finally, the full-time plan exposed a political conflict that grew out of the different material conditions of practitioners and academics. The AMA sought to control medical education as a vehicle for controlling entry into the profession and thereby medical care itself. The scientific medical school faculty, on the other hand, thought that *they* should control medical care. Medical scientists, remarked a prominent British physiologist in 1914, ought to "remodel the whole system so as to fight disease at its source. . . . Surely it is a time when those who have laid the scientific foundations for the new advances should take counsel together, assume some generalship, and show how the combat is to be waged."[25] The Rockefeller philanthropists clearly sided with the medical scientists and cast their weighty fortune with the armies of academe.

Behind the passion of the AMA's attacks were the realizations that the position of medical faculty would no longer be a lucrative supplement for private practitioners *and* that the full-time clinical faculties' main loyalties would be to medical schools and not the organized profession. Elite practitioners would now have to choose *either* a grand income *or* a respected teaching and research position. But even more important to the strategy for controlling medical education, the full-time plan, by reducing the clinician's income and monopolizing his loyalties and material interests in the medical school, would cut the clinical faculty off from private practitioners. Instead of linking together the interests of the elite practitioners with those of the medical schools, full-time clinical faculty would help separate the medical schools from the organized private practice. The full-time plan would reduce the power of the organized profession—in particular, the AMA and its Council on Medical Education—within the medical schools.

Of course, things were different in the 1910s from the way they had been at the turn of the century. The profession's reform strategy had accomplished much of what it set out to do: it had established scientific medicine as the ascending model of medical practice and education, it had reduced the number of schools considerably and thereby the output of new physicians, and it had secured supportive legislation and licensing laws. But the plan had just begun to work, physicians' incomes and prestige were rising, and the end was not in sight. Medical schools were still considered key to the strategy and to continued control by the organized profession of its own material conditions. And the AMA leadership was not about to let that control slip from its grasp. The profession launched a campaign to discredit and oppose the full-time plan.

Selling the Full-Time Proposal

Dr. Welch, an astute medical politician, anticipated the furor the plan would provoke. Four years before Mall suggested the idea to Flexner, Welch had called for reforms that would allow clinical department heads to "devote their *main* energies and time" to teaching and research "without the necessity of seeking their livelihoods in a busy outside practice and without allowing such practice to become their *chief* professional occupation."[26]

When the GEB proposed to fund full-time organization of Hopkins' clinical departments, Welch faced the dilemma of mediating the interests of the laboratory science faculty with those of the clinicians. Welch asked the GEB to allow some exceptions to the full-time rule, enabling the university president or "some other responsible authority" to permit some full-time, salaried professors to keep their consulting fees. The Board adamantly refused to allow any exceptions.[27]

The laboratory faculty unanimously endorsed the plan, but, Flexner later recalled, "there was a rift among the clinicians."[28]

Within two years Welch won sufficient support from clinical faculty. Lewellys Barker, the Hopkins professor of medicine who had publicly advocated the full-time plan in 1902, stood in the way of its implementation at Johns Hopkins. He chose "gold" over "glory" and resigned his professorship, agreeing to become a "clinical professor," drawing a small salary from the medical school but being able to devote most of his time to a lucrative private practice. In his place, Dr. Theodore Janeway gave up his chair at the College of Physicians and Surgeons and an elite practice in New York to become the first full-time professor of medicine in the United States. William Halsted was named professor of surgery and Charles Howland, professor of pediatrics. In October 1913 Welch formally applied for the grant, accepting the condition that the full-time clinical faculty at all ranks—assistant professor to professor—would "derive no pecuniary benefit" from any professional services they rendered. The GEB immediately voted its approval and a grant of $1.5 million.[29]

Three months later the GEB decided to devote all its funds in medical education to "the installation of full-time clinical teaching." Flexner had been hired to administer its program in medical education, and he applied himself with his usual energy.[30]

Within a year Welch reported that "the full-time system is a great success" at Hopkins.[31] Halsted and Howland found the system to their liking, but Janeway resigned his position in 1917 to return to private practice in New York. He was dissatisfied with the full-time arrangements, he wrote in a widely publicized journal article, both because "outside engagements" had been a major source of clinical knowledge to him and because he and his family were used to a higher standard of living than he could afford on his salary. It was "unnatural and repugnant to the patient's sense of justice," he said with great sympathy for his patients, "that a consulting physician should not receive the usual fee for such service."[32]

In 1919 even Osler backed off from his opposition. He asked Welch to use his influence to persuade the GEB to "help McGill start up-to-date clinics in medicine and surgery." Osler made it clear that he did not favor the full-time scheme, but he believed it was now necessary at the Canadian school because "new conditions have arisen" that would leave McGill behind the other first-class schools that had instituted full-time teaching in medicine and surgery.[33]

Over the next few years the GEB voted more than $8 million from its general funds for similar reorganizations on a full-time basis of the medical schools at Washington University of St. Louis, Yale, and the University of Chicago. Applying its matching grant policy, these funds represented several millions more in support for the reforms. Between 1919 and 1921, Rockefeller, Sr. contributed $45 million to the General Education Board specifically for medical education.

The first appropriation from this special fund was a grant of $4 million to Vanderbilt University to make the Nashville medical school a model for the South. The GEB considered Nashville its "strategic point" in the South and Vanderbilt the institution that would lead the drive to improve Southern "public health and industrial and agricultural efficiency."[34] By 1960 the GEB gave Vanderbilt, its major white university in the South, a total of $17.5 million for medical education. Meharry Medical College, the Board's model Negro medical school and one of only two that Flexner had argued should survive, received less than half the sum given to the white institution.[35] Despite its relative stinginess toward black medical education, the Board firmly believed that scientifically trained black doctors were necessary to improve the health of blacks, protect the health of neighboring whites, and provide an elite and unrebellious leadership for the black population. Through its annual grants to Meharry it exerted substantial control and even instituted full-time teaching in medicine and surgery in the 1930s, with approved white faculty members in charge and a hand-picked white president.[36]

The board used its $45 million to foster, if not force, acceptance of the full-time plan at the major medical schools in the country. But not all the schools were won over as easily as Hopkins.

Boston Brahmins Resist

Harvard staunchly refused to accept the full-time plan. In 1913, while negotiating the details of the Hopkins grant with Welch, the GEB invited the Harvard Medical School to apply for a grant to place their clinical departments on a full-time basis. The debt-ridden medical school sought a windfall through subterfuge. The faculty asked for $1.5 million to reorganize all its clinical departments "on a satisfactory university basis." The clinical professors would "devote the major part of their time to school and hospital work," but they could still collect fees from their private patients, whom they would see in offices provided by the teaching hospital. This proposal was hardly consistent with the GEB's by then well-known interpretation of "full-time."[37]

The opposition to the strict full-time policy was led by two powerful members of the Harvard clinical faculty: Harvey Cushing, a renowned neurosurgeon and chief of surgery at Peter Bent Brigham Hospital (a Harvard teaching hospital), and Henry A. Christian, former dean of the medical school. Cushing and Christian, like other members of Harvard's clinical faculty, had lucrative private practices that they refused to give up. They felt it was enough for the clinical faculty to devote themselves to working in the teaching hospital and "to confine their professional activities within its walls." In return, they wanted to accept fees from "patients who might consult us during hours as we felt justified in setting aside for this purpose." Committed though he was to academic medicine, Cushing even offered his resignation to Harvard President Lowell. But, as Cushing undoubtedly knew, Lowell considered the famous surgeon more important to Harvard's academic reputation than the $1.5 million endowment.[38]

Gates and Flexner continued to press for full-time comitments, turning down Harvard's proposals during several years of negotiations. In addition to their ideological commitment to full-time, the GEB members had a pragmatic incentive for pushing it as quickly and widely as possible. Harvard and other schools that allowed their medical faculty to keep their consulting fees were raiding the faculties of schools that adhered to the GEB's policy. In 1921 David Edsall, dean of the Harvard medical school, tried to lure Charles Howland, the Johns Hopkins pediatrician, with the same salary he was getting at Hopkins plus consulting fees from private practice. Flexner had to help Hopkins upgrade their facilities as an inducement to keep Howland there.[39]

Harvard was able to resist the full-time plan because of its reputation as a leading medical school and because its clinical faculty were too prominent in Boston's ruling social circles to be easily dismissed. Already by 1900 the Harvard medical faculty boasted that it controlled "probably more clinical material than any other one school in the country."[40] Such powerful medical figures were also physicians to the Boston upper class, and by virtue of their earnings, and in many cases their births, they were themselves members of the city's very class-conscious upper crust. It took such Brahmins to refuse to surrender their consulting fees in the face of the GEB's compelling offer, particularly when the school's accounts were heavily in the red.

Fear and Trembling in the Board Room

Meanwhile, Charles Eliot, the illustrious former president of Harvard and a trustee of the GEB, carried the battle into the GEB's board room. Eliot argued that "great improvements in medical treatment have in recent years proceeded from men who were in private practice."[41] Eliot went on to argue not merely for Harvard's latest proposal but for a complete reversal of the full-time policy and the binding contracts imposed by the GEB on universities accepting its beneficience. How could the insistence of the GEB on full-time be reconciled with its theoretical hands-off policy, he asked rhetorically. Eliot reminded the Board that it had pledged itself not to interfere with the running of a recipient institution, "except as regards its prudential financial management." Yet the board was making its strict interpretation of full-time clinical organization the condition of a grant. "This condition does not seem to me consistent with what I have always believed the wise and generally acceptable policy of the Board," Eliot diplomatically concluded.[42]

Eliot's argument fell on receptive ears. The Rockefeller philanthropies were under fire from groups, individuals, government commissions, and newspapers spanning a considerable portion of the contemporary political spectrum—from "trust busting" Progesssives and populists, to militant trade unions, to the growing Socialist party. The U.S. Commission on Industrial Relations criticized much of capital's relations with the working class and attacked the Rockefeller and Carnegie foundations' policies for being "colored, if not controlled, to conform to the policies" of the country's major corporations, which are themselves controlled by a "small number of wealthy and powerful financiers."[43] The attacks on unrestricted capital accumulation, the hostility to foundations and the Rockefeller programs in particular, and the increased support for radical and socialist working-class movements greatly impressed the men of the Rockefeller philanthropies.

General Education Board member George Foster Peabody, a New York banker, feared that the rising tide would force the government to assume all support of educational institutions (robbing the foundations of their power and influence) and would also lead to "economic legislation which shall preclude the acquisition of surplus wealth" (the end of capitalism itself). Peabody preached caution in the face of such challenges.[44] Charles Eliot feared the outcome of class conflicts, but he believed the best defense were the programs the foundation had already undertaken:[45]

> We need not imagine that the process of accumulating great fortunes
> . . . is going to continue through the coming generations. . . . The
> evils which I look forward to with dread in the coming years of the
> Republic are injustice inflicted on those who have by those who
> have not, and corruption and extravagence in the expenditure of
> money raised by taxation. Against such evils I know no defense ex-
> cept universal education including the constant inculcation of justice
> and goodwill.

Gates himself feared possible "confiscation" of wealth, but he had faith in the strength of capitalism to survive. "The recognition of the right to earn and hold surplus wealth marks the dawn of civilization," he noted in 1911.[46]

Gates favored standing fast on the principle of private control of wealth and opposed any special defensive strategies. When the president of the Rockefeller Foundation, George Vincent, drafted the annual report for 1917, Gates suggested removing a new self-limiting policy statement. Among other points, the new policy precluded the Foundation from "supporting propaganda which seek to influence public opinion about the social order and political proposals." Vincent defended the statement on the ground that "the one thing that the opponents of foundations seem most to resent is that attempt to control public opinion."[47] It was hoped that the formal statement denying the charges would be accepted by the public as a verdict of innocence.

Fear Undermines the Full-Time Policy

GEB members feared that the full-time contracts would be seen by the public as another example of private capitalist control of essentially public institutions. Visions of more public attacks and restrictive legislation undermined support for the full-time policy within the Board.

Anson Phelps Stokes, who succeeded Peabody as the voice of caution on the GEB, counseled against imposing the full-time policy through contracts. "It is not a question of whether we are right or wrong in our opinions," he explained. The full-time plan itself was not an issue. In fact, he thought it was a commendable program.[48]

> But it is a question of whether or not we can . . . afford—in view of public opinion and our great wealth as a board—to be imposing, or at least requiring, detailed conditions regarding educational policy in medicine in elaborate contracts which can only be amended with our consent. . . . Personally, I think this policy unwise and fraught with serious dangers.

Contracts between the GEB and the medical schools uniformly included a clause specifying that if the full-time plan "shall, without consent of the said General Education Board, be abandoned, substantially modified or departed from, the said university will, upon demand of said Board, return said securities or any securities representing their reinvestment."[49]

Stokes's fear that the contracts would become public knowledge was prophetic. While Eliot, Howell, and the medical faculty at Harvard could be counted on to keep a gentlemanly silence about their conflict with the GEB, the more volatile president of Columbia, Nicholas Murray Butler, was not adverse to airing the conflict. Under Flexner's hard-nosed leadership, the GEB offered Columbia a substantial grant, but only if the university took more decisive control of the medical school, dismissed the reigning dean and clinical faculty while instituting the full-time policy, reduced the student enrollment in the medical school, and took more complete control of Presbyterian Hospital as a teaching facility.[50]

After lengthy negotiations between Butler, Flexner, and representatives of the Presbyterian Hospital trustees, Butler rejected the proposals as "so reactionary and so antagonistic to the best interests of the public, of medical education and of Columbia University, that they will not, under any circumstances, be approved by us."[51] The Presbyterian Hospital trustees, led by philanthropists Edward S. Harkness, W. Sloan, and H. W. deForest, had favored creating a new medical center and had supported all the conditions the GEB was demanding. In 1911 Harkness had given Presbyterian Hospital $1.3 million to encourage them to tighten their bonds with Columbia, giving the medical school exclusive teaching privileges in the hospital and control over Presbyterian's medical staff.[52] Angered at Butler's rejection of the proposals and his support for the existing practitioner-faculty, the hospital trustees voted to sever all ties with the Columbia medical school.[53]

Negotiations continued while the Carnegie Foundation entered the fray in 1919. The Carnegie Foundation joined with the GEB and the Rockefeller Foundation to offer $1 million each toward building a new medical center for Columbia and endowing its faculty. Yet the GEB held out for complete fulfillment of their policy on full-time.[54] Henry Pritchett, of the Carnegie Foundation, could see no reason for such obstinacy. "It is quite true," he told Flexner, "that certain of the professors are allowed to take a small consulting practice. . . . That is not 100 percent fulfillment, but I should say that it was comparable to the claims of Ivory Soap to be 99.44 percent pure."[55]

Pritchett was not only uncommitted to complete subordination of the medical faculty through a strict full-time policy, he also, and perhaps more viscerally, feared attacks on the foundations and the recipient universities. "Such a contract binding a university to a fixed policy laid down by the giver of money seems to me a dangerous thing," he complained to Wallace Buttrick, president of the GEB. "If these contracts were made public, I am sure it would bring down on all educational foundations no less than on the universities themselves severe criticism. It seems to me a dangerous policy for those who administer trust funds to adopt."[56]

The standard response of the GEB officers to such criticisms of their full-time plan contracts was that "the policy was proposed to us by the trustees and medical faculty of the University and that the terms of the contract were such as they themselves asked for."[57] According to this fiction, it was Dr. Welch who proposed the full-time plan to the GEB. "We have never asked any institution to adopt the plan," Buttrick claimed. "The Hopkins proposal in all particulars came from Doctor Welch."[58] This self-serving posture was supported by carefully worded statements in letters, personal contacts, and even the contracts themselves. Flexner and others orally and informally made known the Board's requirements, but they were always careful that any written proposals came from the institution. The painstaking, almost nit-picking negotiations with the Columbia medical school faculty, President Butler, and trustees of the university belie the GEB's claims that it had "no fixed policy regarding medical education" and never attempted to influence the internal policies of universities.[59]

After continued resistance by Harvard and Columbia, public disclosure of the binding contracts, public criticism by the medical profession, and a long history of attacks on corporate philanthropy, the Board in 1925 altered its contracts and thus its full-time policy. Eliot had continued his attacks within the Board meetings right up to the time of his resignation in 1917, charging the group with interfering in the internal affairs of Harvard by demanding full-time organization as the price of an endowment grant. Anson Phelps Stokes carried on the fight to do away with binding contracts and the GEB's narrow definition of full-time.[60]

Window Dressing: Gates Defeated

Although the clamor for abolition of foundations, or at least their severe restriction, had abated with the demise of Progressivism, the entry of the United States into World War I, and the repression of radical and socialist movements following the war, a majority of GEB trustees feared a resurgance of such attacks. "Some day the power of the 'dead hand' will again be the subject of political, if not popular, discussion," warned Thomas Debevoise, legal counsel to the Board.[61]

Debevoise prepared the arguments to support the majority of the trustees in their fight with Flexner and Gates. First, it was important for the Board not to *appear* to control recipient institutions. "It will hurt the reputation of the Board if it attempts to direct the operation of the objects of its bounty," Debevoise argued. Secondly, binding contracts were *unnecessary* to keep the universities in line. "Most of the schools which receive money from the Board come back at least a second time, and the possibility of their needing additional help should lend all the inducement necessary to make them follow the ideas of the Board."[62]

On 26 February 1925 the Board voted, with Gates adamantly dissenting, to authorize a contract with the University of Chicago that required full-time clinical faculty to receive no fees for patients seen in the university's teaching hospitals but allowed them to "continue to engage in the private practice of their professions outside of the University's Hospitals." The contract also allowed the university's board of trustees to make "such modifications and changes by the University in future years as educational and scientific experience may . . . justify."[63]

The final defeat for Gates and Flexner came later that year. At the end of September the executive committee of the GEB voted to modify the original contracts with Johns Hopkins, Vanderbilt, Washington (St. Louis), and Yale universities to allow the boards of trustees to compromise the full-time provision, if they desired. Gates specifically asked to have his negative vote recorded.[64] He took his defeat at age seventy-two as a personal attack and a political blunder. Actually, the policy change was a minor one, a question of tactics rather than strategy.

But in 1925 Gates was a strategist from another era. Although a loyal manager himself, Gates was a product of early corporate capitalism's rugged individualism who never adapted to corporate liberalism's trust in the state and other bureaucratic organizations run by professionals and managers. He did not realize how fully academic medicine was already the instrument of foundation and capitalist interests.

Dependent on outside funding for its capital and operating expenses, medical education could be guided by whoever footed the bill. The GEB and Rockefeller Foundation efforts to institutionalize full-time clinical departments had their effect, even with the resistance and the final defeat of binding contracts. Of the $13 million in medical school operating expenses in 1926, the largest amount—42 percent—went to salaries of full-time faculty. The Commission on Medical Education reported that in the twelve years since the GEB launched its program with Johns Hopkins, the largest single increase in budgets was "for salaries and other expenses in the clinical divisions, particularly in those schools which have placed the clinical departments on a university basis."[65]

Although tuition fees increased to pay for the changes—in 1910, 81 percent of the medical schools charged *less* than $150 per year, while in 1925, 85 percent charged *more* than that in fees—they could not increase beyond the willingness of the middle classes to pay them. Nevertheless, by 1927 more than one-third of the annual income of medical schools still came from tuition fees. Income from endowments was, by the mid-1920s, the second largest source of income and meant the difference, for most medical colleges, between making it as a class "A" school or not making it at all.[66] The influence of the General Education Board and the Rockefeller Foundation were profound.

The full-time plan was an entering wedge, the first thrust of a continuing struggle by corporate philanthropy to control medical education and medical care—to establish the principle that society's needs, as defined by the corporate class, would prevail over the medical profession's interest. It was the first attempt on a large scale to rationalize medical care in the United States. Gates saw clearly the potential value of academic medicine: doctors subordinated to the university, the university controlled by men and women of wealth, and academic physicians researching the causes of disease and eliminating those causes at their microbiological source. All these relationships and functions would ensure that academic doctors, unlike their practitioner colleagues, would serve the needs set before them and not some competing professional interest.

Notes

1. Some examples of this literature include Elliot Friedson, *Profession of Medicine* (New York: Dodd, Mead, 1970); Elton Rayack, *Professional Power and American Medicine* (Cleveland: World Publishing, 1967); and Gerald Markowitz and David Rosner's article in this volume. On medicine as social control, see also Talcott Parsons, *The Social System* (New York: Free Press of Glencoe, 1951), pp. 428-79; Howard B. Waitzkin and Barbara Waterman, *The Exploitation of Illness in Capitalist Society* (Indianapolis: Bobbs-Merrill, 1974); Barbara Ehrenreich and Deirdre English, *Complaints and Disorders: The Sexual Politics of Sickness* (Old Westbury, N.Y.: Feminist Press, 1973); and Ivan Illich, *Medical Nemesis: The Expropriation of Health* (New York: Pantheon, 1976).

2. See Vincente Navarro, *Medicine Under Capitalism* (New York:

Charity, Science, and Class

Prodist Publishers, 1976), for a discussion of the relationship of the state in capitalist society to health and medical care.

3. For a fuller discussion of the developing relationship between the medical profession and the capitalist class, see E. Richard Brown, *Rockefeller Medicine Men: Medicine and Capitalism in America* (Berkeley: University of California Press, 1979).

4. Rosemary Stevens, *American Medicine and the Public Interest* (New Haven: Yale University Press, 1971), pp. 68-69; see also Richard H. Shryock, *American Medical Research, Past and Present* (New York: Commonwealth Fund, 1947), pp. 96-97.

5. Diana Long Hall, "The Rockefeller Foundation and the Creation of American Sex Endocrinology, 1921-39," paper presented at the American Academy of Arts and Sciences annual meeting, 27 February 1976.

6. Abraham Flexner, *Medical Education in the United States and Canada* (New York: Carnegie Foundation for the Advancement of Teaching, Bulletin No. 4, 1910). See also Howard S. Berliner, "A Larger Perspective on the Flexner Report," *International Journal of Health Services* 5 (1975): 573-92; and Markowitz and Rosner in this volume.

7. On the impact of the Flexner report, see Rosemary Stevens, *American Medicine,* pp. 68-69; William G. Rothstein, *American Physicians in the Nineteenth Century* (Baltimore: Johns Hopkins University Press, 1972), pp. 292-94; Markowitz and Rosner, in this volume; and Robert P. Hudson, "Abraham Flexner in Perspective: American Medical Education, 1865-1910," *Bulletin of the History of Medicine* 46 (1972): 545-61.

8. *Annual Report of the General Education Board,* 1919-1920, 1928-1929.

9. Abraham Flexner, *Abraham Flexner: An Autobiography* (New York: Simon and Schuster, 1960), pp. 109-10; Raymond B. Fosdick, *Adventure in Giving, The Story of the General Education Board* (New York: Harper and Row, 1962), pp. 154-55; and A. Flexner to F. T. Gates, 24 June 1911, GEB files, Rockefeller Foundation Archives (hereafter cited as "RFA").

10. A. Flexner, *Autobiography,* pp. 110-11.

11. Ibid., pp. 112-13; Fosdick, *Adventure,* p. 157; A. Flexner, "From the Report on the Johns Hopkins Medical School," GEB files, RFA.

12. See George W. Corner, *A History of the Rockefeller Institute, 1901-1953* (New York: Rockefeller Institute Press, 1964), p. 94; and S. Flexner and J. T. Flexner, *William Henry Welch and the Heroic Age of American Medicine* (New York: The Viking Press, 1941), p. 304. The policy was established before the hospital opened in 1910.

13. F. T. Gates, "Concerning Private Gifts to States and a Medical Policy," Memo to the General Education Board, 26 February 1925, Gates collection RFA (hereafter, "Private Gifts").

14. J. D. Greene to Dr. Henry A. Christian, 30 November 1914, GEB files, RFA.

15. Gates, "Private Gifts."

16. For descriptive history of the full-time plan's origins, see Flexner and Flexner, *Welch,* pp. 297-314, 320-28.

17. Richard H. Shryock, *The Unique Influence of the Johns Hopkins University on American Medicine* (Copenhagen: Ejnar Munksgaard, 1953), p. 19.

18. Florence R. Sabin, *Franklin Paine Mall, The Story of a Mind* (Baltimore: Johns Hopkins Press, 1934), especially pp. 29, 127-33, 203, 261, 264.

19. *Journal of the American Medical Association* 35 (1900): 501.

20. Victor C. Vaughan, "Reorganization of Clinical Teaching," *Journal of the American Medical Association* 64 (1915): 785-90.

21. Quoted in Sabin, *Mall*, p. 270.

22. Fosdick, *Adventure*, p. 160.

23. Stevens, *American Medicine*, p. 96.

24. Arthur D. Bevan, "Report of the Council on Medical Education," *Journal of the American Medical Association* 65 (1915): 110-11.

25. Benjamin Moore, "The Value of Research in the Development of National Health," *Popular Science Monthly* 85 (1914): 366.

26. Quoted in Ilza Veith and Franklin C. McLean, *Medicine at the University of Chicago, 1927-1952* (Chicago: University of Chicago Press, 1952), p. 22.

27. William H. Welch, "Report on the Endowment of University Medical Education," 1911, copy in GEB files, RFA.

28. A. Flexner, *Autobiography*, pp. 114-15.

29. Welch's letter to GEB, quoted in Fosdick, *Adventure*, p. 158.

30. Ibid., p. 159.

31. William H. Welch to Simon Flexner, 5 December 1915, GEB files, RFA.

32. Quoted in S. Flexner and J. T. Flexner, *Welch*, p. 326. Janeway's article was "Outside Professional Engagements by Members of Professional Faculties," published in Nicholas Murray Butler's journal, *Educational Review* 55 (1918): 207-19.

33. Quoted in S. Flexner and J. T. Flexner, *Welch,* pp. 326-27.

34. A. Flexner to H. S. Pritchett, 27 March 1919, correspondence with GEB, Carnegie Foundation files.

35. Fosdick, *Adventure,* p. 328.

36. Ibid., p. 180.

37. Fulton, *Cushing,* pp. 383-84; Fosdick, *Adventure,* p. 163.

38. Ibid., p. 163; Fulton, *Cushing,* pp. 377-84.

39. A. Flexner to W. Buttrick, 7 May 1921, GEB files, RFA.

40. "Reasons Why the Harvard Medical School Offers the Best Opportunities for Surgical Scientific Work," by "members of the Surgical Department," attached to letter H. P. Bowditch (?) to John D. Rockefeller, Jr., 31 October 1900, Record group 2, Rockefeller Family Archives.

41. Eliot quoted in Fosdick, *Adventure,* p. 163.

42. Ibid., p. 164. On the Rockefellers and their relations with others, see Peter Collier and David Horowitz, *The Rockefellers, An American Dynasty* (New York: Holt, Rinehart, and Winston, 1976).

43. Commission on Industrial Relations, *Final Report* (Washington, D. C.: Barnard and Miller Print, 1915), pp. 116-19. See also James Wein-

stein, *The Corporate Ideal in the Liberal State, 1900-1918* (Boston: Beacon Press, 1968), pp. 172-213.

44. G. F. Peabody to F. T. Gates, 5 November 1911, Record group 2, Rockefeller Family Archives.

45. C. W. Eliot to F. T. Gates, 27 March 1914, Gates collection, RFA.

46. F. T. Gates, memo to himself or the Board, (n.d., but apparently November 1911), Record group 2, Rockefeller Family Archives.

47. George E. Vincent, *The Rockefeller Foundation, A Review for 1917* (New York: Rockefeller Foundation, 1918), p. 8; F. T. Gates to G. E. Vincent, 20 March 1918, and G. E. Vincent to F. T. Gates, 25 March 1918, Record group 1, Program and Policy File, RFA.

48. Fosdick, *Adventure,* p. 164.

49. Ibid., p. 164.

50. Catherine Lewerth, "Source Book for a History of the Rockefeller Foundation," (typewritten ms., bound in 21 volumes, Rockefeller Foundation Archives, c. 1949), pp. 5,116, 1,119-21.

51. Quoted in ibid., p. 5,115.

52. *Annual Report of the General Education Board, 1920-1921* (New York: GEB, 1922), p. 22.

53. Lewerth, "Source Book," pp. 5,115-16.

54. H. S. Pritchett to Wallace Buttrick, 11, 24 February 1919, Correspondence with GEB, Carnegie Foundation files.

55. Pritchett to Flexner, 10 June 1925, Correspondence with GEB, Carnegie Foundation files.

56. H. S. Pritchett to Wallace Buttrick, 11 November 1919, Correspondence with GEB, Carnegie Foundation files.

57. W. Buttrick to H. S. Pritchett, 21 November 1919, Correspondence with GEB, Carnegie Foundation files.

58. W. Buttrick to Harry Pratt Judson, president of University of Chicago, 26 December 1914, GEB files, RFA.

59. Correspondence regarding Columbia University medical school, 1917-1920, GEB files, RFA; W. Buttrick to H. S. Pritchett, 21 November 1919, Correspondence with GEB, Carnegie Foundation files.

60. C. W. Eliot to W. Buttrick, 24 April 1917, GEB files, RFA; A. P. Stokes to A. Flexner, 10 March 1925, GEB files, RFA. Stokes was always wary of public criticism that the GEB was attempting to control educational institutions with its grants (cf. A. P. Stokes to W. Buttrick, 29 January 1917, GEB files, RFA.).

61. T. M. Debevoise to F. T. Gates, 7 October 1925, GEB files, RFA.

62. Ibid.

63. Minutes of the GEB, 26 February 1925, GEB files, RFA.

64. Minutes of the GEB Executive Committee, 30 September 1925, GEB files, RFA.

65. Commission on Medical Education, *Supplement to the Third Report* (New Haven: Office of the Director of the Study, May 1929), p. 58.

66. Commission on Medical Education, *Supplement,* pp. 58-59.

BARBARA G. ROSENKRANTZ
and MARIS A. VINOVSKIS

9   *Sustaining "the Flickering Flame of Life": Accountability and Culpability for Death in Ante-Bellum Massachusetts Asylums*

Although death may be a fact of life, the logical and inevitable terminus of grave illness, or the final chapter of a long life, the occasion of death requires special recognition and explanation. Contemporary Americans are concerned about the economic, social, and emotional costs of life-prolonging medical interventions. They are also troubled by consequences for the dying and the bereaved of institutional death, dying among strangers, or in an aseptic hospital environment that estranges familiar associations.

Even when the hospital is looked on as a source of comfort, death within its walls challenges both its image as a safe haven for the sick and the therapeutic skills of the physician. Personal grief may be assuaged through religious faith or through remembrance that misery has ended for a loved family member; yet these comforts have rarely obviated the haunting sense that the outcome might have been otherwise. Commitment of a person to the hospital, however determined, may arouse guilt in family members when death rather than recovery occurs, and guilt may well awaken suspicion that improper care or neglect has has-

We are indebted to Mary Vinovskis for programming the data and to Terry Hill for research assistance. Funds for this research were provided by NIH Grant No. LM 02355-03. A draft of this paper was presented at the Social Science History Association Meeting at Ann Arbor, Michigan, October 1977. We wish to thank Gerald N. Grob for comments made at that time.

tened death. Whatever the circumstances, when hospitalization terminates in death, a measure of extra responsibility devolves upon the medical authority charged to support life until the very end and to account for the particular moment that marks the extinction of pulse-beat and breath.

In ante-bellum Massachusetts, medical superintendents of asylums for the insane responded to deaths in their hospitals in ways that revealed anxieties about their institutions' reputations and reflected professional responsibility for their patients. Physicians in these institutions had more intimate day-to-day contact with their patients than was customary in most medical care of the period. In part, this was because the favored treatment of insanity accentuated particularly intrusive management of patients' behavior; this led to the use of hospitals for the treatment of insanity to a far greater extent than for treatment of other diseases.[1] Before the Civil War each state had built at least one public asylum designed to house patients of every social class and condition of mental derangement. The physical structure of these institutions was carefully planned to meet the individual's and society's needs; the internal regimen was organized for no more than 250 inmates. Private asylums, usually of considerably smaller size but otherwise intended to function in a remarkably similar manner, were more numerous.[2] Altogether less than a half of those persons identified as insane at any specific date were inmates of these asylums. Commitment was frequently advised, however, when physicians were consulted, or when viewed as medically desirable for the afflicted, compatible with the duties of families and friends, and advantageous for community agencies in the case of the dependent lunatic.

The determination to commit a person to one of these asylums was arrived at with the expectation that recovery would follow treatment. For most persons committed before the Civil War to the McLean Asylum, a private hospital that opened in 1818 (a total of more than 4,500 admissions), or the Worcester State Hospital which opened in 1833 (a total of more than 6,000 admissions), death was not anticipated in the hospital. Although many insane appeared moribund on entering these hospitals, a far larger proportion were discharged as "recovered" than as "unimproved" or "died." Yet the physicians who were in charge felt compelled to address both personal and

156

institutional culpability for mortality within the asylum. This article is confined to that topic: The explanation of mortality within the walls of two Massachusetts hospitals, the McLean Asylum in Somerville and the Worcester State Hospital, by their medical superintendents in the decades preceding the Civil War. We focus on the physicians' acknowledgements of their professional responsibility for the health of these institutions and the inmates. Our sources are the published annual reports of superintendents and trustees, journal articles, the mortality statistics gained from hospital records, and the relatively sketchy accounts of events immediately preceding death and the death scene itself found in the case records of patients.[3]

Support for the organization of asylums for the insane in the United States in the first decades of the nineteenth century was partly influenced by earlier English and French examples; inspired by humanitarian concerns and new concepts of insanity, Old World efforts to alleviate perpetual custody of the mad had led to some noteworthy institutional reforms.[4] When the insane were separated from other incarcerated persons, solicitous treatment and medical management had restored hopeless maniacs to rational behavior. Physicians at the McLean Asylum and the Worcester State Hospital turned to these experiences from abroad to confirm their own belief that insanity was a disease that would respond to enlightened treatment. The origins of insanity were believed to be both physical and moral or psychological. The victims of this pathology could be found among all classes and in most cases, when promptly treated, could be returned to useful lives. McLean and the Worcester State Hospital were among the first American institutions to establish the formal environment required for moral and medical treatment.

The superintendent-physicians appointed by trustees of both these hospitals were charged to select assistants, supervise admission of patients, and manage all contingencies so that their new institutions would meet the expectations fostered by European example and American perfectionist sympathies. They took on these heavy responsibilities with some assurance that their previous professional experiences had earned the confidence leading to their appointment. They anticipated attracting patients quickly. McLean was intended to serve about 100 insane persons, largely those who could pay for the cost of board and treatment. In contrast, the State Hospital, although making provisions for paying patients, was expected to receive up to 250 insane already dependent on local and state support and who would otherwise have been neglected at home or in jails and poorhouses.

Intent on constructing a regimen of discipline, Dr. Rufus Wyman, the first superintendent at McLean, Dr. Samuel B. Woodward, the first at the State Hospital, and the physicians they recommended to succeed them, were eager to admit patients most likely to be responsive to treatment. In the first part of this article we will indicate characteristic modes through which the physicians addressed the uneasiness that death within the asylum engendered and distinguish three issues which appeared to ensure accountability without incurring fault. In the second part we will discuss the superintendents' attitudes towards reporting and comparing mortality statistics and show how these data were interpreted in the light of contemporary information and apprehensions. In a brief examination of asylum mortality rates within the context of other characteristics of the total patient population we will return, at the close of the article, to an assessment of the social burden carried by explanations of death within these two institutions designed for cure.

Superintendents' Explanations of Mortality in Asylums

Though our analysis of death will be confined to the experience within these hospitals, the attitudes of the superintendents and their patients were certainly influenced by more general behavior and perceptions associated with death and dying in ante-bellum America. Ideally, we would have liked to compare responses to the moribund within the hospitals with the care of the dying and attitudes toward death in the rest of society. Unfortunately, there is not enough substantive research available on death and dying in nineteenth-century America to permit such a comparison at this time.[5]

Although superintendents were not eager to accept long-standing cases of insanity, there is little indication that this reluctance was initially motivated by fear that such patients would die in the hospital. Physicians were interested in demonstrating the efficacy of their therapy. Treatment was believed most effective when begun soon after the appearance of the symptoms of insanity, and families were warned that chronic cases were not likely to benefit from treatment in even the best institution. In general, medical superintendents and trustees of asylums argued persuasively that removal of the insane from their homes and from family influences was a prerequisite for recovery. But since the hospital environment was seldom viewed as desirable for the sick in families with domestic help and financial means, it was imperative that asylums for the insane be viewed in a different light if they were to be patronized by the well-to-do.

Although we do not know whether death among strangers was viewed as particularly fearsome, we do know that asylum doctors needed to defend the salubrity of their institutions, even though some patients died while in their care. It was not enough to record instances when death was the expected outcome of long suffering, although brief entries in asylum case books such as "death comes to his relief" testify to this conclusion. Both McLean and Worcester case books record that the dead were claimed by friends and relatives in most instances, and frequently at McLean there are records of autopsies performed before burial took place. We know also that at McLean the dying were sometimes attended by next of kin and that chapel funeral services were on some occasions conducted at the institution itself, both for those who died as inmates and for the recently discharged. Accepting death and memorializing the dead were, no doubt, much affected by the particular condition of the deceased as well as by sentiments originating outside the hospital.

Accounting for death within the asylum was, nevertheless, clearly a matter of special concern. The inevitability of death rather than absolving the superintendents of responsibility, required them to identify those conditions that were most hazardous to the life of the insane and were most frequently associated with insanity. The problem of accounting for deaths was compounded by the fact that death rates of insane patients were higher than those of the general population. With annual death rates in the asylum averaging around 10 percent and sometimes soaring to even higher levels, the superintendents felt compelled to justify the elevated mortality levels (see Figure 9-1).[6] The three most frequently cited reasons were the physical debility of entering patients, the increased likelihood of

159

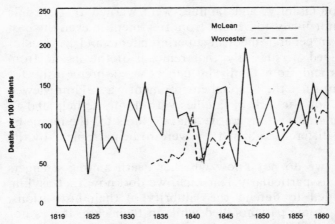

Figure 9-1. Number of Deaths per 1,000 Patients at McClean Asylum (1819-1860) and Worcester State Hospital (1833-1860).

death of the insane due to association of insanity with a fatal disease, and the continuous threat of epidemics imported from outside the asylum.

As soon as Worcester State Hospital opened its doors in 1833, Dr. Samuel B. Woodward, its superintendent, also expressed concern that jails and poorhouses would disgorge their inmates on the pretext of insanity and fill the hospital with persons who were unlikely to benefit from therapy. Though particularly wary of the criminal whose customary habits would interfere with the order required at the hospital, Woodward understood nonetheless the institution's social obligation to admit individuals directed there by state and local authorities. But even as he acknowledged the responsibility of a public institution, he warned that this charge might obstruct his assigned task. For Woodward, the burden of death in the hospital was evidence of the miscarriage of his mission. Beginning in his first report to the trustees, Woodward advised the public to expect a larger number of deaths "than in other institutions of the kind" since, unlike private asylums, the State Hospital was obligated by law to accept all persons "sent by the courts."[7]

It is not surprising, therefore, that Woodward's attention to the problem of mortality, was usually very closely linked to fluctuations in mortality at the hospital. When mortality levels were low, as in 1835-1837, he did not devote much effort to accounting for the deaths of patients. When there was a sudden rise in mortality, as in 1838-1839, he explained and justified these deaths by emphasizing the unhealthy condition of the patients on admission. He often resorted to another theme as well: that families sent their dying relatives and friends to the hospital because they were too troublesome at home.

Woodward's successor, Dr. George Chandler, also lamented the fact that debilitated patients entered the hospital and quickly died, frequently within the first month. Yet in some ways Chandler was less concerned about justifying the mortality levels at Worcester. Perhaps it was because high mortality levels in these institutions had been well established by the time he assumed office in 1846. Instead, Chandler was disturbed by the incurability of many debilitated and often chronic patients who might not die within the first month, but might remain at the hospital with little hope for successful treatment. Chandler, like Woodward, was especially vigilant about maintaining the therapeutic function of the hospital; he railed against sending patients there who would either die immediately or stay indefinitely.

In 1851, after three years of high mortality, Chandler expressed discouragement without explicitly noting that the proportion of deaths to total number of patients in the hospital's census did not significantly exceed previous records. The statistical report for that year, 39 deaths among 704 patients, was followed by the observation that mortality will always be large "when patients are not removed after a short residence." "Maniacal exhaustion" shares a place with "Consumption" and "Apoplexy and Palsy" as the most frequent causes of fatality, and Chandler writes that "Insanity with many is but one of the symptoms of a general breaking up of the physical constitution. The incurable, if not removed, must sooner or later be included in our bills of mortality."[8]

The response to death at the McLean Asylum was markedly different at the outset. Dr. Rufus Wyman, the first medical superintendent, found almost no occasion to remark directly on the extent of mortality at that institution.[9] In the absence of statistics from a comparable American hospital, there was little reason to compare mortality levels at McLean with those of

161

the insane hospitalized abroad, in Massachusetts jails, or in poor-houses. McLean had a distinct task with reference to a specific population, primarily the insane with the means and inclination to afford the best care. After the Worcester State Hospital was established, Wyman's successor, Dr. Luther V. Bell, repeatedly argued that the special resources and obligations of a private asylum such as McLean left little reason for comparison with other institutions. Perhaps there was an obvious incentive for his view since the annual death rate for the smaller population at McLean was usually higher than at Worcester and fluctuated more sharply from year to year. Bell made fewer references to deaths in the hospital than Woodward and Chandler and apparently did not consider the mortality rate a hazard to McLean's reputation. Acknowledging that patients were often sent to the asylum so debilitated that death must inevitably follow, McLean's superintendents assumed some of the responsibilities of a hospice to the dying.

Although successful treatment was anticipated for the same reasons given at Worcester and other ante-bellum institutions for the insane, in admitting the moribund, McLean established a pattern of respectability. Bell scarcely bothered to justify the number of deaths reported in any specific year, though he noted that "with hardly an exception" these were "subjects broken down in general decay, old age or epilepsy . . . ." Instead he called attention to the asylum's policy of admitting the insane without regard to general health at the moment of commitment. At the same time, when Bell instituted a policy of discharging the chronically insane who demonstrated little chance of recovery, he was willing to provide beds for the dying so long as space was available. Even when pressed for accommodations, he reported that

> it has been considered a duty to advise the reception indiscriminately of all cases for which application has been made, without inquiring as to any other point of their derangement. . . . In conformity to this principle there has been placed under our care, several whose state of health was such as to render speedy death almost certain, as well as many whose cases were hopeless from their long duration, or complicated with the imbecility of old age or epilepsy. The fact that six out of the eight cases of death, occurred within the first month of the sufferer's residence, presents a key to the character of many of our admissions.[10]

162

Since a substantial number of the deaths in both institutions were of aged and "decayed" insane persons, different policies toward admission of the elderly inevitably are reflected in the response to death itself. The greater latitude in the rhetoric about admission of the aged to McLean, not always followed by the actual commitment of a large number of elderly patients, could be interpreted as a reflection of a more sympathetic attitude toward the patient threatened by death.[11] A more sober explanation is found in the social ties with patients' families; the presence of a relative at the bedside of the dying was not uncommon. Furthermore, the cause of those debilities that sent aged moribund patients to institutions was often diagnosed as merely simulating insanity and antedating hospitalization. The implication of culpability was thus removed from the superintendent, leaving a more lenient attitude toward reception of the dying to be determined by other considerations.

General debility was only one of the conditions that threatened the life of the insane. At a period when diagnosis and prognosis were the most respected tools of the physician, medical superintendents conscientiously recorded and evaluated the influence of all diseases upon the insane. It was clear that insanity was aggravated and more likely to have a fatal outcome in the presence of other illnesses. Insanity, furthermore, often led to death from ordinary diseases that might otherwise have been self-limited. Bell's caution about the consequences of comparing statistics from different institutions also led him to warn against too precise assignment of the cause of insanity. This practice, intimately associated with the collection of statistics, led to "giving an apparently mathematical and certain aspect to facts, so involved in doubt, so complicated and vacillating, that they really have nothing like fixedness and certainty."[12]

Yet the connection between prevailing medical theory and specific concepts about the management of the insane resulted in a mode of interpreting disease in the insane as reason for their unusual vulnerability to death. The generally labile nature of inflamation in which benign fevers were transformed into malignant maladies, was exaggerated in the insane. In the insane an ordinary illness took on different symptoms:

> The diseased fancy perverts their position or their relative importance, and in cases arrived at or approaching demency or loss of

mind, the altered manner, aspect, and habits, are nearly all indications which are externally presented of even greater disorganizing changes. In the form of exhaustion referred to, many of the sufferers sink much as those in extreme age; as if the lamp of life were exhausted, without the machinery being subverted. In others again, the form that it takes is the loss of all resiliency, all recuperative energy in the combat with affections not ordinarily fatal. A slight influenza, or a little gastric derangement, appears to have lost its self-limited, self-remedying character, and involves the energies of life, notwithstanding the employment of curative means.[13]

Marasmus, that "universal failure of the powers of life, admitting of no place in the ordinary nosological catalogues," by general agreement headed the list of diseases that threatened the life of the insane. This pathology and its near associate, consumption, led to general wasting away and "emaciation of the whole system."[14] Indistinguishable from the debility associated with melancholia and senile dementia, fatality from these interactive causes hovered over the asylum in a form that forecast death even when fatality was not specifically anticipated.

Patients admitted with delirium are properly considered in this category too. Sometimes the superintendents turned to the accusation of improper commitment in accounting for death of the febrile patient. A more common assessment at the State Hospital than at McLean was: "Many cases have incurable diseases when they enter the hospital." The difficulty of differential diagnosis once stated, Woodward points the finger at the committing agency: "Frequently a case is brought to our care, with delirium of fever, instead of insanity, in which the journey aggravates every symptom, and death immediately follows."[15] At McLean a patient who dies within a week of admission is recognized "upon examination . . . and before the parties who brought her had left the house" to be very feeble and in a critical condition.[16] In these cases the burden was twofold: first, that the death might be improperly charged to neglect or other failure of treatment; second, that a person stricken with a disease from which recovery was possible would suffer needlessly and ultimately die because he had been disturbed and taken from home. Fatal outcome in the case of a fever was almost proof of improper diagnosis for Woodward, who argued that "deaths from acute diseases, affecting persons recently insane are extremely rare with us."[17] Commitment in such cases un-justly taxed the resources of the hospital and imperiled the patient. Febrile diseases were not uncommonly mistaken by family, friends, and even physicians for the symptoms of in-sanity. Hospital mortality, then, was unreasonably elevated by the tendency to commit without cautious differentiation among symptoms. In effect, this argument revealed the unpleasant possibility that deaths often occurred through the undue haste of the committing agency. At McLean there is less overt rejec-tion of the feverish patient who is destined to swell the mor-tality list. Instead, the trustees are assured in the superinten-dent's report that "it almost never has happened that a removal of a sick and hopeless case has been made."[18]

Epilepsy, the second most fatal illness of the insane, pro-vided another easily identified and acceptable model for an-ticipated death. Woodward's reputation for successful treat-ment of this disease did not apparently cast doubt on the legitimacy of deaths from this cause. Woodward had attracted the admiration of physicians who were members of the Associa-tion of Medical Superintendents of American Institutions for the Insane with the implication of curing epilepsy through therapy with stramonium, nitrate of silver and sugar of lead. This may have laid the foundation for a perceptibly tolerant attitude toward epileptic patients at the Worcester State Hospital, where "kind and conciliating" management was counseled as late as 1850, despite the great risk of death in epileptics.[19] At both Worcester and McLean these patients were viewed as acceptable for admission even though cure was not expected and death was the likely outcome of sudden seizures. Epilepsy was intimately associated with the cause and symptoms of in-sanity itself. Yet once more responsibility for the origin of this disease preceded the hospital environment and regimen.

It turns out that the threat of multiple deaths from epidemic disease should have provided superintendents in both institu-tions the best opportunities for demonstration of their effective role in abating mortality. Both institutions were able to show resistance to the ravages of cholera that swept the nation in the late 1840s. Bell gratefully celebrated complete freedom from that dreadful scourge despite the fact that Boston was afflicted "and many of the most intense and virulent cases of this epi-demic were in the village between us and the city." Chandler noted that "that mysterious disease" left the State Hospital un-scathed except as it lowered "the tone of physical health." In general, superintendents used these occasions to fashion a reservoir of confidence that addressed death indirectly by certi-fying the soundness of the physical environment and the archi-tectural provisions at the hospital. Free of the "mimotic dis-orders which have been thought to attend the train of the Asiatic Cholera," Bell went further: "If there were premonitory indications of the effects of a malarious atmosphere among us, their actual nature was lost sight of in the facility of their yield-ing to medical agents."[20] At other times, when a siege of some other epidemic disease within each institution took its toll, the superintendents noted that patients were less affected than at-tendants and their own immediate families.

But annual fluctuations in mortality were not necessarily a stimulus to accountability. Worcester superintendents, ever sen-sitive to perturbations that were actually smaller and less fre-quent than those at McLean, showed no inclination to take ad-vantage of this comparison. On the other hand, they looked to this circumstance as a means of advertising that the hospital protected its inmates against local deleterious influences. When mortality statistics showed a rise in 1838, the next year's *Annual Report* emphasized that the institution was excellently equipped with a ventilation system providing warm air that assisted in resisting diseases.[21]

At McLeans neither a sharp increase nor a drop in deaths ap-pear to have required or invited interpretation. The one excep-tion came with a distinct rise in mortality in 1847, which was partly due, according to Bell, to the low number of deaths the previous year. Both Bell and the McLean trustees demonstrated a proclivity to account for elevated mortality entirely in local terms and disregarded this opportunity to assess their situation with reference to others. The trustees reported 70 cases of dis-ease and 12 deaths among the 170 patients. Crediting the "un-remitting efforts of the officers and attendants" with the responsibility for the low case fatality rate, both the superinten-dent's and the trustees' reports looked inward, gaining confidence from the fact that there was only one among the dead "of whose ultimate recovery there was the slightest hope." While the recovery rate among the patients was such as "to excite sur-prise and gratitude," the epidemics insulated McLean from the need to defend its healthy environment and arrangements.[22] Bell showed suprisingly little anxiety about public response to fluctuations in mortality at the asylum.

While both institutions were able to place epidemic disease in a context that improved the image of the hospital as a fortress against untoward illness leading to unwarranted deaths, on the whole the superintendents and trustees in neither institution seem to have taken full advantage of their fortunate escape from cholera. In the different responses to illness and death among attendants and members of their own families lies a suggestion of the obstacles.

Chandler remarks that at Worcester the insane had largely been immune from three cycles of measles because they "lived in a more uniform temperature and were less exposed to the vicissitudes of the season" than hospital aides and even than his own daughters.[23] But, having otherwise diminished hospital responsibility for deaths by asserting the unavoidability of mortality when incurable and debilitated persons were committed, there was less opportunity for associating prevention of death with the possibility of cure from insanity, the ultimate defense of the hospital regimen. And at McLean, where trustees memorialized Bell's unswerving devotion to the asylum's inmates in the face of grief over deaths of his young son and daughter in 1847, the sense was overwhelming that the patients' deaths came despite the best medical attention. Accommodation to death is here couched in conventional sentiments sent from the trustees to Bell and his family: "May their grief be soothed by the gentle ministry of time,—by the hallowed memories of the past, the high duties of the present, and the sacred hopes of the future!"[24] Thus they recognized the function of the hospital community to support the bereaved, more than to prevent the unavoidable.

Both institutions, having established a rationale that accounted for deaths from specific causes, saw the integrity of their responsibility best defended in this way. Deaths of vulnerable individuals, not the statistics of institutional mortality, were at issue. If this meant that escape from epidemic disease received less credit than it might otherwise, it also meant that the traditional defense of institutional objectives through statistical demonstration took on a different role when the data of mortality were involved.

The Superintendents' Use of Mortality Statistics

Most of the superintendents' accounting for the high mortality levels in their institutions was devoted to explaining the difficult constraints under which they operated. Though they might have preferred not to reveal or discuss the number of deaths in their hospitals, the superintendents felt obligated to do so in their annual reports. The usual reporting procedure for mortality was to record the number of deaths during the past year. In some years there would be an extended discussion of the number, causes, or rate of deaths, while in other years the data would be cursorily reported. Very rarely were there any efforts made to analyze the aggregate mortality data beyond the presentation of simple descriptive statistics.

The possibility of invidious comparisons with other institutions was always present unless the objectives of asylums were first well established. Foremost in the mind of those superintendents who were obliged to provide space for former inmates of jails and poorhouses was the dilemma of maintaining public support through relieving the towns and the Commonwealth of dependent individuals whose incurable disease or intractable behavior was not accessible to hospital therapy. The conventional categories of reporting did not lend themselves to the intricate adjustments required under these circumstances.[25] Reporting deaths, along with other conditions of patients on discharge, scarcely left room for consideration of the special risks incurred when treating the insane. Moreover, these hospitals, both private and public, were unique institutions.

Comparison with other institutions invited compromise and ignorance of important differences. It was tempting, nonetheless, to cite statistics from abroad when they showed that mortality "in the British and French Hospitals is much greater than in ours, amounting to 22 to 25 percent, while in ours is less than 7 1/3 percent." More often the variability of these data made this procedure hazardous.[26] American superintendents also avoided comparison with other local receptacles. When mortality rates at the Massachusetts State Prison were shown to be considerably lower than at the State Hospital, Chandler responded immediately.

It by no means follows from this, however, that the diet and mode of life in the Hospital are less salubrious than in the prison. The prisoners are mostly men of vigorous organization, and at a period of life during which mortality is least. In most of our patients, the original stock of vitality was probably small, in almost all it was sadly impaired before admission. Many brought here a poor flickering flame of life, which would have soon been extinguished in the gusty world without, but which is now carefully tended, and will lick up the last drop of oil ere it dies in the socket.[27]

It is more surprising, however, that Chandler and his assistants at Worcester never noted publicly when their annual mortality rates were lower than those at McLean. Perhaps they did not want to offend any of their powerful supporters of the well-established private asylum since their endorsement might be necessary later. One can also surmise that the advocates of moral and medical therapy were glad to be distracted from attention to mortality since in their view it begged the more important question of misuse of their facilities. The mode of reporting aggregate data deprived them, however, of identifying specific factors that would have shown a rather admirable record. Focusing on the patient's characteristics that restricted the chance to cure insanity, they denigrated the meaning of mortality rates and rejected, on other grounds, the implications of the data they felt obligated to publish.

One of the common analyses used by superintendents to report the relative healthiness of their hospitals was to calculate the ratio of the number of deaths to the average number of patients during that year. Using this procedure, we can calculate the annual number of deaths per 1,000 patients at the McLean Asylum and the Worcester State Hospital. Overall, the number of deaths per 1,000 patients was considerably higher at McLean (111/1,000) than at Worcester (89/1,000). Even if we recalculate the McLean data for the years 1833-1860 in order to make them chronologically comparable to those at Worcester, the difference remains the same (110/1,000 against 89/1,000).

There were considerable fluctuations in the annual death rates in the hospitals, ranging from a low of 37/1,000 to a high of 203/1,000 at McLean and a low of 56/1,000 to a high of 134/1,000 at Worcester. Not only was the range in deaths greater at McLean than at Worcester, but there was generally greater annual variation in death rates at McLean. In part, some

169

of the greater fluctuation in annual mortality at McLean is due to the smaller number of patients in that institution; but even for those years in which the average number of patients in the two hospitals are more comparable, it still appears that McLean experienced a greater fluctuation than Worcester.

Though McLean usually had higher annual death rates than Worcester, its patients were slightly less likely to die there than those in the State Hospital. While 12.1 percent of the patients at McLean died while under asylum care, 13.2 percent of those at Worcester died before discharge. The percentage of patients who at some time were recorded as dying within the hospital is very different than the percentage of patients who die in a given year, for the latter figure includes many other factors such as the rate of turnover in the hospitals and the length of time the patients remain in that hospital. The superintendents of the hospitals could only consider the annual number of deaths since they had no way of knowing the eventual fate of the patients they admitted. Therefore, while McLean appeared to have a higher death rate than Worcester, based on the ratio of the annual number of deaths to the average number of patients in those hospitals, patients at McLean were actually less likely to die there than those at Worcester. The most important thing to note, however, is that the overall percentage of patients dying in those two institutions was almost identical.

While there were great variations in the annual death rates at McLean, there was no long-term secular trend. At McLean the decade of the 1830s had the highest death rates, while the 1820s and 1850s had the lowest death rates. There was a definite upward trend in death rates, however, at Worcester. While annual death rates there averaged 71/1,000 during the 1830s and 76/1,000 during the 1840s, they rose to 100/1,000 during the 1850s. By the 1850s the average annual death rates at Worcester were almost as high as those at McLean (100/1,000 vs 109/1,000).

While in retrospect we can evaluate these mortality patterns as intimately tied to the demographic characteristics of the population received at each institution, contemporary superintendents were more concerned with identifying the patient characteristics that were related to the defense of their institutions' primary justification and achievement, the successful treatment of insanity. When compelled to report statistics of mortality, the superintendents focused on explanations of the association of death with the etiology and nature of insanity. While they subjected the specific kinds of insanity related to fatality to scrupulous analysis, they neglected to identify those factors such as age, marital status, and by whom the patient was committed, which might have influenced the risk of death no matter what manner of insanity was involved. No doubt because the superintendents were so deeply committed to generating and preserving their institutions' reputations, they simply neglected the value of differentiating some of the important determinants of mortality other than disease that characterized their patients on admission and in the period of hospitalization that, for some, terminated in death.

The analysis of annual death rates is a very crude procedure since that ratio can be influenced by a wide variety of factors. In an effort to explore these hospital deaths in more depth, we assembled individual-level data on the characteristics of the patients at McLean (1818-1859) and at Worcester (1833-1859). A few of the patients were excluded from this analysis because of missing data on at least one of the variables; the total number of cases used from McLean was 2,941 and 5,837 from Worcester.[28]

Our analysis attempts to explain the factors associated with a patient dying in the hospital (hence our dependent variable is dichotomous: 1=patient died in hospital/0=patient did not die in hospital). Since we want to consider more than one independent variable at a time, we used multiple classification analysis.[29] A variety of different independent variables were considered, but our final list included only six factors—the age of the patient at admission, their length of stay in the hospital, by whom were they committed, the decade in which they were committed, the gender of the patient, and their marital status. Ideally, we would have like to include other independent variables such as the physical condition of the patient upon entry, but that information is not available in the general registers or the case books at either McLean or Worcester. Although our analysis is certainly limited by the variety of factors employed, our six independent variables can tell us a lot more about the likelihood of a patient dying than could be gleaned from the

171

crude statistics on mortality presented by the superintendents in their annual reports.

One of the most obvious determinants of the likelihood of dying in these hospitals was the age of the patient when admitted. The superintendents were aware of the fact that the older patients were more apt to die than the younger ones; they even complained that some of the elderly patients were sent to the hospitals to die because their friends and relatives did not want to care for them during their last days. Our analysis confirms that the age of the patient at admission was a very important factor in determining the chance of death in the hospital (see Figure 9-2). Although, as noted earlier, patients admitted at ages cester were slightly more apt to die than those at McLean, it is interesting to observe that of the patients admitted at ages seventy and above, those at McLean were much more likely to die than those at Worcester. In part, this is a reflection of the differences in policy toward the aged patients. Although McLean was not eager to receive elderly patients for whom there was little hope of recovery, once these individuals were sent to the hospital the superintendents were willing to have them stay there, even if it simply meant that they would eventually die in the hospital. The superintendents at Worcester, however, tried to discourage elderly patients from remaining long enough to die. They sought to have them transferred to some other state institution or returned to their family and friends once it became apparent that they were incurable.

Since the superintendents in both hospitals were anxious first of all to encourage admission of patients likely to benefit from treatment, moribund patients were implicitly subsumed in the category of inappropriate admissions. Medical superintendents paid more attention to the deaths of those who died shortly after admission than to the likelihood that chronic patients would eventually raise mortality rates. Death of chronic patients, that is those whose insanity was of long standing and who were therefore discouraged from entering the hospital because they would not ever demonstrate the efficacy of treatment, was not the subject of separate statistical accounting. Because we wanted to see whether the risk of death increased for patients who remained in either institution more than a year, we ran a multiple classification analysis first with the patients' ages on admission and then with ages at discharge.

Among patients hospitalized less than a month, the percentage of deaths was quite high. In part this is a reflection of the fact that most patients were not discharged from the hospitals in less than a month since the therapy offered them usually required a longer time period. But even taking this into consideration, the first month in the hospital was still relatively dangerous. At McLean 3.4 percent of all patients died during the first month (or 27.7 percent of all deaths occurred in the first month), while at Worcester 2.1 percent of all patients died during the first month (or 15.9 percent of all their deaths). Thus, the superintendents of the hospitals were correct in noting the relatively high death rates among newcomers to the hospital.

If a patient remained in the hospital for more than a year, the risk of dying also increased (see Figure 9-3). This is partly a reflection of increased age and also because with increased age patients became more vulnerable to fatal disease. Although the superintendents, particularly those at Worcester, discussed how the burden of chronic patients damaged their record of successful treatments, they paid less attention to the consequence of chronicness for mortality rates. Death of those individuals committed to a public institution may well not have seemed so critical to the institution's reputation as continued expensive support of dependent, incurably insane persons.

This question is closely related to a problem that did receive attention from the superintendents. While Bell and his successors at McLean were more willing to give comfort to the dying than Chandler and those who followed him at Worcester, physicians at both institutions were convinced that there was a general tendency to shirk personal and social responsibility for the helpless aged and moribund. Since the cost of hospital care was higher than maintenance in local almshouses and jails, there should have been less incentive to commit the dying insane who were public charges. Yet the mortality rates of those committed by state courts and town authorities were no higher than those of the insane brought to hospitals by relatives and friends (see Figure 9-4).

The fact that only a small portion of the total patient population in either institution died within the first months after commitment reinforces our conclusion that superintendents had an exaggerated view of the extent to which institutions were relied

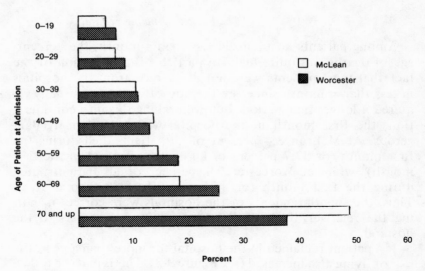

Figure 9-2. Adjusted Percentage of Patients Who Died, by Age of Patient at Admission.

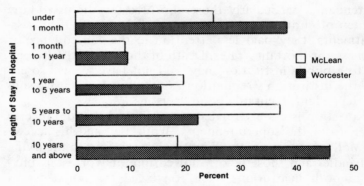

Figure 9-3. Adjusted Percentage of Patients Who Died, by Length of Stay in Hospital.

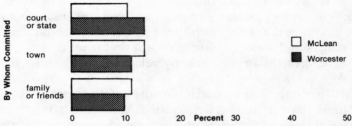

Figure 9-4. Adjusted Percentage of Patients Who Died, by Who Committed Them.

upon to care for the dying. A longitudinal analysis of the rate of mortality in both asylums during the ante-bellum years shows only a slight increase over time in the probability of dying after admission to the hospital (see Figure 9-5). While long-term custody increased the number of deaths occurring annually, the superintendents were mistaken in their conclusion that the purpose of the institution was being subverted by the dying.

Although there was discussion about the role that gender played in susceptibility to insanity, women being considered more vulnerable than men by some authorities such as Edward Jarvis, there were no statistics to demonstrate their greater risk of hospital death.[30] Similarly, though domestic troubles were identified as the cause of insanity more often in women than men, marital status was not even recorded in reporting mortality. Women and men were admitted to both hospitals in approximately equal numbers, and we found little difference in death rates association with gender (see Figure 9-6).

The marital status of the patient was related to the likelihood of death, but not very strongly. Before controlling for the other factors, we found that single patients were the least apt to die in the hospital while patients who were widowed or separated were the the most at risk. These results are not unexpected since single patients tended to be among the youngest while widowed or separated patients were likely to be among the oldest patients.

When we controlled for the effects of the other variables, such as the age of the patient upon admission, the least likely to die were still the married patients while the most likely to die were those who were widowed or separated—though the differences among patients by their marital status had narrowed considerably (see Figure 9-7). The results might indicate that married patients had a slight advantage over other patients because of the emotional and material support they may have received from their families. The stress associated with being widowed or separated may have made it even more difficult to recover from insanity. Though the relationship between marital status and the probability of dying is not particularly strong, the results are consistent with those from present studies that find married individuals to be less likely to experience disorders and difficulties than those who are widowed, divorced, or separated.

175

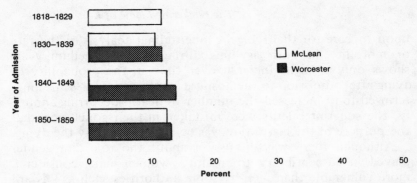

Figure 9-5. Adjusted Percentage of Patients Who Died, by Year of Admission of Patient.

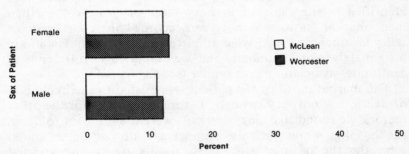

Figure 9-6. Adjusted Percentage of Patients Who Died, by Gender of Patient.

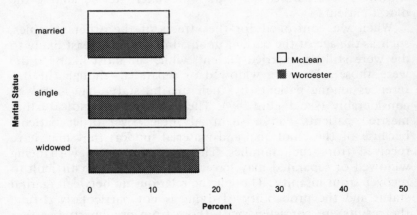

Figure 9-7. Adjusted Percentage of Patients Who Died, by Marital Status of Patient.

Conclusion

Mortality rates in these two ante-bellum asylums assuredly reflected the precarious health of the inmates. The death of patients inevitably raised doubts about commitment, treatment, and the adequacy of care. Where the blame would fall, how responsibility would be deflected or assumed, reveals much about the image that the superintendents had of themselves and their institutions, which were so heavily influenced by this personal image.

Protecting the reputation of their institutions, the superintendents sought both solace and authority through explanations of death that fit their medical knowledge. Many patients were destined to die because of their previous condition of health and the deprivations they had suffered at home or in other institutions. Some were believed to be especially vulnerable because of the nature of insanity itself, while others were seen as liable to die because mild diseases became malignant as a result of lesions of the brain or negligent behavior characteristic of insanity. Whatever the link between insanity and fatal illness, the institution itself was defended.

Within the general rubric of defense, differences in arguments made by the superintendents of McLean and Worcester reflected their sensitivity to the expectations of their constituents. Woodward, Chandler, and his successor, Dr. Merrick Bemis, saw Worcester State Hospital's very existence threatened by mortality statistics that might raise doubts about the purpose and efficacy of their institution. The "statistical point of view" is valuable only "when drawn from a long period of time, and from a large number of patients, and with full understanding of all the circumstances which may have influences upon them." Chandler prefaces his accounting for the year 1854 with the graphic reminder that "a picture of the Hospital edifice is more or less pleasing according as it is taken from one or another point of view, so an account of its sanatory condition will be more or less favorable according as it may be taken from one or another statistical view."[31] For most of the ante-bellum period the Worcester superintendents took the stance that elevated mortality came about through influences beyond their control and wishes, primarily a consequence of social policies that unwisely sent them patients whose condition precluded cure.

177

Deaths were but one sensitive indicator of the obstacles under which they labored.

McLean superintendents, on the other hand, were generally in a position to be more receptive to the moribund. Their obligation included provision of respite to the families of dying patients through care and comfort in the final days of waning life. The superintendent was the central figure at McLean. With greater latitude than that enjoyed by the physicians at Worcester, Wyman, Bell, and Tyler could show compassion without concern that their asylum's purpose would be perverted through the dark images associated with custody and death. Only when the dying threatened to take places from more treatable patients was there warning about improper commitments. Institutional integrity was protected by both opportunities to evaluate the desirability of expansion and decisions based on responsibility internal to the organization and structure of authority in the hospital, rather than by reference to larger community duty.

In a very real sense the social environment not only threatened patients' lives but shaped the lives of these institutions as well. McLean, with greater resources, retained its image as a therapeutic asylum that could provide space and comfort for the dying as well. Worcester State Hospital, however, took on a mocking semblance of the role that once it had rejected. By 1865 the superintendent adopted words that previously had been associated only with McLean. Speaking of the dying patient, he reported that "while they incommode the general order, and give by their decay and death a melancholy character to the department to which they belong, they are doubtless proper subjects for the care and concern of the hospital."[32] Ironically, this sentiment was not tied to the cult of curability that once had been Worcester's primary hope but, rather, to the gradual acceptance of the mission of custody for the incurably insane. Despair made death more reasonable and provided room for the dying.

Notes

1. Charles E. Rosenberg, "The Therapeutic Revolution: Medicine, Meaning and Social Change in 19th Century America," *Perspectives in Biology and Medicine* 22 (1977): 485-506. Rosenberg, "And Heal the Sick: The Hospital and the Patient in the [sic] 19th Century America," *Journal of Social History* 10 (1977): 428-47. For the most recent comprehensive description of public institutions for the mentally ill in this period, see Gerald N. Grob, *Mental Institutions in America: Social Policy to 1875* (New York, 1973).

2. For a discussion of popular and scientific ideas about insanity, see Norman Dain, *Concepts of Insanity in the United States 1789-1865* (New Brunswick, N. J., 1964). For a more specific description of therapy employed, see Eric T. Carlson and Norman Dain, "The Psychotherapy That Was Moral Treatment," *American Journal of Psychiatry* 117 (1960): 519-24. For a history of the Worcester Hospital, see Gerald N. Grob, *The State and the Mentally Ill: A History of Worcester State Hospital in Massachusetts 1830-1920* (Chapel Hill, N.C., 1966). There is no published history of the McLean Asylum.

3. This article is part of an extensive study of asylums drawn from institutional and patients' records. In addition to the records cited here, our research includes manuscript records of the Hartford Retreat (now the Institute of Living) and the Institute of the Pennsylvania Hospital. To facilitate our research and encourage others to use these resources, we have coded data on the socio-demographic characteristics of patients—the histories, admissions, diagnoses, treatments and discharges of inmates for computer-based files which can serve in part as indices to the records deposited in these hospitals' archives and libraries. The Worcester records for this period are located in Holmes Hall (the Rare Book Collection) of the Francis A. Countway Library of Medicine (Harvard). For information on research in progress, see the authors.

4. Physicians and laymen concerned with treatment of the insane went to England and the European continent to visit institutions and learn about their arrangements. Not every method used abroad was believed adaptable to New World patients; for instance, American physicians were generally not convinced that the absence of physical restraints advocated in England would be wise. American physicians who studied the literature from abroad, however, agreed that commitment of the insane to special institutions was desirable. The account of institutional organization which first won admiring attention was Samuel Tuke, *Description of the Retreat, an Institution Near York for Insane Persons of the Society of Friends* (York, England, 1813). Philippe Pinel's *Nosographie Philosophique* (Paris, 1898) and *A Treatise on Insanity,* trans. D. D. Davis (Sheffield, England, 1806), shaped a diagnostic and therapeutic philosphy that was congruent with treatment in a hospital environment.

5. Most recent work on death in early America focuses on the seventeenth and eighteenth centuries though it usually does make some reference to the changing attitudes toward death and dying during the first half of

the nineteenth century. For example, see David E. Stannard, *The Puritan Way of Death: A Study in Religion, Culture, and Social Change* (New York, 1977); Peter Gregg Slater, *Children in the New England Mind: In Death and in Life* (Hamden, Conn., 1977).

There are some recent essays on death in nineteenth-century America which suggest some of the critical issues associated with death and dying in ante-bellum America. Lewis O. Saum, "Death in the Popular Mind of Pre-Civil War America," in *Death in America,* ed. David E. Stannard (Philadelphia, 1975), pp. 30-48; Ann Douglas, "Heaven Our Home: Consolation Literature in the Northern United States, 1830-1880," ibid., pp. 49-68; Stanley French, "The Cemetery as Cultural Institution: The Establishment of Mount Auburn and the 'Rural Cemetery' Movement," ibid., pp. 69-91; Jean Bertrand, "From Skull and Crossbones to Winged Cherubs: Perceptions of Deaths in America, 1845-1885" (Senior Honors Thesis, University of Michigan, 1976); Maris A. Vinovskis, "Angels' Heads and Weeping Willows: Death in Early America," in *Themes in the History of the Family,* ed. Tamara K. Hareven (Worcester, Mass., 1978), pp. 25-54.

6. Death rates for Boston in this period fluctuated between 20 and 30 per 1,000, see *Historical Statistics of the United States,* 3rd series, part I (1975). For an interpretation of mortality data in Massachusetts, see Maris A. Vinovskis, "Mortality Rates and Trends in Massachusetts before 1860," *Journal of Economic History* 32 (1972): 184-213.

7. *First Annual Report of the Trustees of the State Lunatic Hospital at Worcester* (December 1833), pp. 53-54. These published annual reports included the superintendents' formal accounting to the trustees and tables of hospital statistics from the current and former years.

8. *Nineteenth Annual Report of the . . . Hospital at Worcester* (December 1851), pp. 53-54.

9. Wyman retired in 1835; he had been in constant attendance at the Asylum since 1818.

10. *Twentieth Annual Report of the Physicians and Superintendent of the McLean Asylum for the Insane, to the Trustees of the Massachusetts General Hospital* (January 1838), pp. 12-13.

11. For an analysis of the underrepresentation of aged among insane committed to asylums, see Barbara G. Rosenkrantz and Maris A. Vinovskis, "The Invisible Lunatics: Old Age and Insanity in Mid-nineteenth Century Massachusetts," in Stuart F. Spicker *et al., Aging and the Elderly* (Atlantic Highlands, N.J., 1978).

12. *Twenty-third Annual Report . . . of the McLean Asylum* (January 1841), p. 12.

13. *Twenty-sixth Annual Report . . . of the McLean Asylum* (January 1844), p. 34.

14. Bell expressed surprise that only two "amongst the more than eighty deaths which are registered" in McLean's first quarter-century were from "phthisis," a disease that would probably be classified as pulmonary tuberculosis today. This low percentage has not been achieved by discharging the terminally ill, "since it has almost never happened that a removal of a sick and helpless case was made." Furthermore, Bell reports that he has "known only two instances where this disease has occurred in

patients after their removal" (*Twenty-sixth Annual Report . . . of the McLean Asylum* [January 1844], pp. 35-36). By contrast, although Woodward ranks most fatal diseases of somatic origin that are exacerbated by insanity in approximately the same order, he finds that a large number die of consumption or phthisis; many times patients arrived at the hospital with the symptoms of this disease (*Sixth Annual Report of the . . . Hospital at Worcester* [December 1838], p. 47). "The little regard which the insane have to prudence and care respecting health, and the frequency of their exposure and privations renders them particularly liable to a class of diseases in no way connected with insanity" (*Ninth Annual Report of the . . . Hospital at Worcester* [December 1841], p. 50). The Worcester Hospital admission registers, however, show that only a very small number were admitted with consumption listed as a cause of commitment (which, of course, in no way contradicts Woodward's observation).

15. *Fourteenth Annual Report of the . . . Hospital at Worcester* (December 1846), p. 52. This complaint of fever terminating in death at the hospital when the patient might have recovered if left at home is one of Woodward's frequent observations.

16. McLean Asylum bound casebook for 1854-56. The patient lived ten days following admission, but the record made after death sounds very much as though she would not have been accepted as a patient if her condition had been accurately assessed from the outset. This would contradict Bell's general observations a decade earlier, and reflects both changing criteria over time and the not remarkable discrepancy between policy and practice.

17. *Thirteenth Annual Report of the . . . Hospital at Worcester* (December 1845), p. 69. Woodward consistently stated that, when the febrile were also in fact insane, they responded to hospital treatment. Somewhat ambiguously, he also frequently asserted that "an institution of the character of this Hospital will always be liable to receive such cases of insanity complicated with other diseases as will swell the catalogue of deaths, and increase its fatality above that of hospitals which have power to reject unfavorable cases" (*Sixth Annual Report of the . . . Hospital at Worcester* [December 1838], p. 46).

18. See note 14.

19. *Eighteenth Annual Report of the . . . Hospital at Worcester* (December 1850), p. 55. This same report states that in epilepsy "little can be done effectually in the way of medical treatment." In slight cases the stramonium cure had "some reputation; in a few cases, unconnected with insanity, a mitigation and a cure even has followed their protracted use. But the instances of recovery are rare."

20. *Thirty-second Annual Report . . . of the McLean Asylum* (January 1848), p. 16. *Seventeenth Annual Report of the . . . Hospital at Worcester* (December 1849), p. 47.

21. *Seventeenth Annual Report of the . . . Hospital at Worcester* (December 1839), p. 78.

22. *Thirty-second Annual Report . . . of the McLean Asylum* (January 1848), pp. 48-49.

23. The measles epidemic commenced with one attendant. "Three suc-

cessive crops of this contagious disease succeeded. Thirteen of our attendants and eight patients, and my two daughters had it." Chandler noticed that the disease was more severe as new victims succumbed, and that the attendants suffered worse than the insane. Fortunately, there were no fatalities (*Seventeenth Annual Report of the . . . Hospital at Worcester* [December 1849], p. 46).

24. *Thirty-second Annual Report . . . of the McLean Asylum* (January 1848), p. 50.

25. Although the asylum registers used a row for each admission in which separate columns listed admission data (including residence on admission and whether the commitment was made by family, court, selectmen, etc.), the column on discharge stated simply "recovered," "improved," "stationary," or "died." Annual reporting of conditions of discharge was made by tabulating the column without reference to data associated with admission.

26. Edward Jarvis, M.D., "On the Comparative Liability of Males and Females to Insanity and Their Comparative Curability and Mortality When Insane," *American Journal of Insanity* 7 (1850): 142-171. *Eleventh Annual Report of the . . . Hospital at Worcester* (December 1843), pp. 35-36.

27. *Twenty-second Annual Report of the . . . Hospital at Worcester* (December 1854), p. 14.

28. During this period there were 4,703 admissions to McLean and 6,407 to the Worcester Hospital.

29. Multiple Classification Analysis is a form of multiple regression analysis with dummy variables which express results in terms of adjusted deviations from the grand mean (overall average) of the dependent variable of each of the various classes of the predictor variables. For example, MCA answers the question: how much of the likelihood of dying in a hospital was associated with the age of the patient after controlling for other variables such as the length of stay in the hospital, the marital status of the patient, and the decade in which he or she was committed? Similarly, it provides an approximate answer to the question: *ceteris paribus,* what is the effect on the likelihood of dying in a hospital of the particular age of the patient? MCA "controls" for other variables by assuming, while it looks at one class of a predictor variable, that the distribution of all other predictor variables will be the same in that class as in the total population, thus "holding constant" their effects. Although traditional multiple regression programs also do this, MCA has three advantages: it does not require variables to be interval variables; it does not require or assume linearity and thus can capture discontinuities in the direction of the association; and finally, it is useful descriptively because it presents the reader with the gross effects of a predictor class, that is, the actual mean of each class, as well as the mean after adjusting for the influence of the other variables.

30. See Jarvis, "On the Comparative Liability," pp. 142-71, and *Eleventh Annual Report of the . . . Hospital at Worcester* (December 1843), pp. 35-36.

31. *Twenty-second Annual Report of the . . . Hospital at Worcester* (December 1854), p. 13.

32. *Thirty-third Annual Report of the . . . Hospital at Worcester* (October 1865), p. 10.

PART IV

DOCTORS, NURSES, AND WORKERS: SCIENTIFIC MEDICINE AND SCIENTIFIC MANAGEMENT

As the health sector has grown in size and complexity, various groups of health professionals and workers have sought, through different means, to gain or retain control over their work. Conflicts often arise between workers, professionals, and the health institutions in this process, during which both the nature of health services and the structure of the institutions are transformed. The articles in this section examine three essential groups in the health sector—doctors, nurses, and non-professional workers—and trace their methods of organizing as the center of health care moved from doctors' offices and private homes into the hospitals.

Gerald Markowitz and David Rosner trace the relationship between medical education and medical reform at the turn of the century. They argue that physicians were concerned with their lowly social and economic status and threatened by the growing importance of hospital-based care. In response, the doctors, in conjunction with corporate foundations, developed new forms of professional control. Susan Reverby is concerned with the changing work relations within the hospital. She posits that the rationalization of nursing work was the result of the interaction between changing nursing professionalization and hospital management paternalism. Leon Fink and Brian Greenberg present a case study of one of the earliest hospital unionization drives. They analyze the relationship between the workers' efforts, the philanthropic paternalistic foundations of the hospital, and the transformation of the institution from a long-term to an acute care facility.

The major question raised by these articles is: What is the relationship between the changing political economy of the health sector and its work force? Is there something particular to the health industry in this process? How are both work and the work force transformed during this development? What determines the forms of organization of professionals and workers and the responses of administrators and trustees? What are the implications of these changes for patient care and the financing of health care?

GERALD E. MARKOWITZ
and DAVID ROSNER

---

10 *Doctors in Crisis: Medical
Education and Medical Reform
During the Progressive Era,
1895-1915*

During the past decade, doctors have been subject to increasing criticism. Some critics, particularly in the early 1970s,
focused on the fact that doctors seemed excessively interested
in increasing their status and acheiving large incomes commen-
surate with high social standing. Recent criticism of physicians
has centered on new, and perhaps more serious, issues. Patients
now question the very authority of physicians, particularly
when new procedures or medications are prescribed without
sufficient explanation. Hospital workers are more likely to resent the physicians' assumed centrality, especially when so
much of health care depends upon them. Finally, doctors are
perceived as a conservative force at a time when changes in
health care delivery seem imperative.

Historians have sought to explain the conservatism of doctors
and their opposition to progressive health measures. They assert that a shift occurred in the medical profession's ideology
and public positions after World War I, when organized medicine began an active campaign against any government involvement in medical care or financing. Prior to 1917, it is held, the
medical profession, and the American Medical Association in
particular, supported national health legislation and therefore
represented a liberal or progressive force in America.

Copyright 1973, Trustees of The University of Pennsylvania. A slightly
different version of this article originally appeared in *American Quarterly*
25 (March 1973), 83-107.

It is said that the chief mechanism used to secure a high status and income for doctors has been the limitation of the number of physicians in America. The prevailing interpretation is that this practice arose during the 1930s as a result of the Great Depression and the consequent economic deprivations suffered by doctors and others. Elton Rayack argues that it is clear that "restriction of the supply of physicians' services was a basic goal of organized medicine during the depression decade." Rayack maintains that earlier twentieth century "restriction on supply . . . seems to have been an unintended by-product of a socially justifiable desire to raise deplorably low standards of medical training."[1] The other standard view is that the Flexner Report of 1910 was a watershed in the reform of medical education. Sponsored by the Carnegie Foundation and written by Abraham Flexner, this document recommended reduction in the number of medical schools and the introduction of science and laboratory-based courses in the remaining schools.[2]

Our examination of the medical profession suggests instead that the origins of its conservatism lie in the early twentieth century, before 1910, and more precisely in the efforts to modernize and reform medical education. These reforms have been described as progressive and liberal, and they were, insofar as they raised standards and combated dangerous quackery. But the campaign to reform medical education had other goals as well. Specifically, it sought to restrict the number of doctors and consolidate medical facilities within certain well-defined lines. The AMA was in the forefront of that effort, and drew its strength from two groups within the medical profession, the private practitioners and the university hospital-based specialist-teachers. These two groups often clashed over policy matters within the AMA, but they united in pushing reform of medical education. Each believed that the economic and social situation of individual doctors and the profession in general was discouraging. In part this arose from the general feeling of crisis that permeated the society during the depression of the 1890s. In addition, physicians and other professional groups saw their status and power being eroded and engulfed by the tremendous growth, consolidation, and control of industrial capitalism. Doctors sought to assure their financial security and power through their own organization and reform of medical education. At the same time, the profession solved a number of internal problems: it consolidated the components of the emerging university-medical school complex and restricted intra-professional competition.

The consolidation of power and restriction of competition in medicine did not occur in a vacuum. Reform in the Progressive Era often incorporated the business models of efficiency and scientific management. Reformers looked to larger units and centralized administration as essential components of their efforts. Such reform was often used by big businessmen and other elite groups in the society to consolidate and secure their power.[3] The "expert" became the key to change in the society. As the business model of efficiency came to replace more personal values, peoples' ability to understand their own conditions and to choose intelligently among various alternatives was increasingly doubted. For example, city governments replaced personal, albeit corrupt, ward bosses and district leaders with efficient, impersonal, "clean" commissioners. Coincident with the rise of the expert, was a shift in "the location of decision-making away from the grass roots, the smaller contexts of life, to the larger networks of human interaction."[4] As a result, federal regulation superceded state regulation. At the same time, however, in much of rural and small town America the older and less organized patterns of life continued.

This was precisely the situation in medicine at the turn of the century. The nineteenth century, individualistic, personal medical care system predominated, with the private practitioner as the bulwark of the system. But at the beginning of the Progressive Era he was increasingly challenged and threatened by a new system and a new type of physician. These physicians were concentrated predominantly in large cities on the East Coast, and they practiced primarily in universities, hospitals, or medical school complexes. It was this latter group that was campaigning for a more scientifically based medicine, and the expansion of the business model into medicine and medical education. One doctor put the issue directly:

> Why should not the group-unit, which is so plainly the chief efficiency factor in industrial and commercial enterprises, be the same in medical practice? Could not small groups of medical men, specializing or semispecializing, achieve far greater results, primarily for the patient and secondarily for themselves? We are constantly confronted with perplexities based directly on the erroneous archaic

notions of medical practice which certain outworn traditions have kept alive. There is too much laissez-faire.[5]

These ideas and policies were pushed with increasing vigor and effectiveness by a new and powerful consolidating force: the foundations sponsored by Rockefeller, Carnegie, and other industrialists. They put all their resources behind the centralization of power and decision-making in medicine and medical education.

Although many of the individualistic private practitioners felt threatened by the growing strength of this medical elite and its powerful allies, they were even more concerned about what they perceived to be the depressed state of the profession. Thus, most of them cooperated with the university-based physician in the effort to reform medicine and improve their condition. Responding to the cry of "organize or perish," private practitioners flocked to join the AMA during the Progressive Era. From 8,400 member doctors in 1900, the AMA jumped to 70,000 by 1910 and represented fully 60 percent of the nation's doctors by 1920. Still, this rapid organization was not an end in itself, but a way to affect state licensing, public health legislation, and medical education.

"Never was the outlook so gloomy," the *Journal of the American Medical Association* (*JAMA*) complained in an 1898 statement of the profession's fears and concerns.[6] In spite of scientific advances, the status, power, and income of most doctors were perceived by the profession's spokesmen as low and inadequate. One doctor, writing in the *Pittsburg Medical Review,* lamented that it was "humiliating to make a comparison of the economic and social positions of our leading physicians and surgeons . . . with leading lawyers and other professional men."[7] The profession was interested in raising its social standing, power, and income. Medicine's official voice, JAMA, declared that "the standing and influence of the medical profession depend on the material success and financial independence of its members."[8]

Many locally based doctors perceived themselves as "poor". Some doctors complained that there was real, as opposed to relative, poverty. In an article entitled "Why is the Profession Poor in Purse?" Dr. C. H. Reed of Toledo, Ohio, recounted a story of "a doctor who was found crying because he was hungry."[9] But the author of an article in *Cosmopolitan* also suggested that the real problem was not starvation or real poverty but, rather, the relative status and income of the physician in relation to other professional groups. The income "of many a medical man," the article stated, "who has spent years in acquiring a medical education is often less than that of an ordinary mechanic,"[10] an unnerving comparison for the "professional" physician.

Other medical spokesmen defined the problem as being a maldistribution of wealth within the profession itself. A few physicians garnered all the riches while the great mass of private practitioners suffered financially. The official journal of the Medical Society of the State of New York complained, "There is a handsome income for a few, a competence for the many, a pittance for the majority."[11] In a rather stinging editorial denouncing this maldistribution of funds within the profession, the *Medical Record* noted bitterly that while the rich doctors may have to "cut off a few of their luxuries in times of stringency . . . the ordinary practitioner . . . suffers in good times and in bad."[12]

Doctors believed that the loss of their income, like the loss of their status, was a comparatively new development.[13] With the advent of various sanitary reforms, antitoxins, protective sera, and increased education, the physician saw mortality rates steadily declining, giving cause to worry that perhaps the actual need for the physician would diminish. Furthermore, the number of non-medical personnel working in the health field had also increased, making certain skills of the private and general practitioner obsolete. In 1880 there were only 15,601 nurses, by 1900 the number had increased to 120,000. The number of midwives also rose, and there were 5,000 osteopaths, 5,000 Christian Scientists, as well as numerous chiropractors and others who were also viewed by the profession as forms of competition.[14]

The overwhelming argument used by physicians to explain their recently incurred poverty was that the profession was "overcrowded." One spokesman claimed that one-third the number of doctors could do the work of all, which would solve the problem of money.[15] Others echoed this point of view. Writing in *JAMA*, Dr. T. J. Happel complained, "The profession is overcrowded, and is becoming more and more so every year."[16]

A near obsession with "overcrowding" developed and was reinforced by a doctor-to-population ratio that was among the lowest in the world. "It has been estimated that it requires one thousand of the population to ensure to a physician a decent living," one doctor wrote, "yet in these United States the average is one physician to 700 or 800 population."[17] The European doctor-to-population ratio was much higher. In Germany, for instance, the proportion was over 2,000 to 1.[18] Confronted by such a disparity, *JAMA* warned "that we must be rapidly approaching the limit of additions to the medical profession if the individual members are to find the practice a lucrative profession."[19]

How to limit the number of doctors became a serious and persistent problem for the medical profession. The *AMA* and its constituent bodies tried to limit the number of doctors through state licensing and control; but the major thrust was through control of medical education and limitation of the number of graduates by lowering the number of existing schools. *JAMA* argued in 1901, fully nine years before the famous Flexner Report, that through the death of old doctors and the increase in population there was "room for nearly 3,300 new doctors each year," but there were approximately 160 medical colleges producing about 6,000 graduates yearly. The *Journal* issued a warning that "the multiplication of doctor-factories has gone far enough in this country. . . . It is not a dignified comparison, that of the medical graduates to the output of a machine shop," it admitted, "but the same principles of political economy apply in a measure to both. Overproduction in either has its bad effects, and we have not the recourse of foreign markets enjoyed by the ordinary manufacturer."[20] Just like the monopolistic corporate enterprises whose organization they copied, the profession sought to restrict supply in order to maintain and increase their price and profits.[21]

Overcrowding, furthermore, was seen as the root cause for a number of ethical "abuses". These included fee-splitting, nostrums, and the use of free hospitals and out-patient clinics by patients who were able to pay private practitioners. The oversupply of doctors led to a "scramble for business by many of its members."[22] The "excessive" number of "regular" physicians was serious enough, but *JAMA* and other leading state journals also fumed at the large number of "irregular" doctors

and "quacks" who further limited the doctors income and status. To Dr. Chaillé, dean of the Medical Department of Tulane
University, "quacks" were "the greatest foe to the medical
profession" because they represented a great "obstacle to the
financial success of the reputable medical practitioner."[23]

The drive by the "regular profession" against osteopathy and
other competing groups was often conducted on the basis of
high moral principles and the quality of medical care. But one
observer urged that such rhetoric should be abandoned. "This
verbiage is all cant, these benefits are incidental, but our opponents take advantage of this muddle of words to make confusion worse confounded. . . . What we really want is effective
protection against the various pretenders to the healing art."[24]
JAMA editorialized: "Overcrowding means treading on each
others toes, scrambling, more or less decorous, certainly not
tending to the dignity of the profession, going far beyond the
bounds of generous rivalry. . . ."[25]

It should be remembered that much of the concern about
"overcrowding" was voiced during the severe depression of the
1890s. During this period few if any of the working-class groups
on whom most local physicians depended could afford to pay a
private practitioner. For much of the population struggling
through that depression, private medical services were an unnecessary luxury. As alternatives to paying private practitioners,
the poor and the newly arrived immigrants often sought care
from one of a number of cheaper sources: the out-patient clinics of hospitals (known then as hospital dispensaries) where
general practitioner and specialist care was available; the public,
medical school, or charity dispensaries, where medical care was
also gratis to the consumer; and from the "lodge" or "club"
where, for a relatively small cost, a physician's services were
guaranteed for a specified period of time. To the private practitioner, consumers using these alternative services were viewed as
lost clients. Furthermore, the private practitioner saw the specialist and the young, newly graduated physicians who were
staffing the alternative care facilities as the perpetrators of the
crisis.

A conflict developed between the individual private practitioner and the physician associated with the growing university
medical school and hospital complexes. The latter increasingly

demanded the consolidation of the existing components of the medical system: medical schools, universities, hospitals, and private foundations. Within this group, and centered among those in the elite, eastern, university medical schools, there arose a movement and a far-ranging set of goals for medical education reform. These reformers wanted to raise the standards of the profession through the elimination of incompetency, the use of scientific methods, and extensive laboratory and clinical experience. Integral to this effort was a simultaneous drive to consolidate the competing institutions of medical education. The reform movement went charging off to battle, adopting as its motto, "Fewer and better doctors." The large university medical schools would be supreme. Smaller medical colleges were to be wiped out or merged with other institutions. Hospitals were to become an integral part of the medical school and to provide the clinical material for medical students. Foundations were to provide the funds for university-based professors to conduct research using, if necessary, the clinical material provided by the hospital.

Elevation of the standard of medicine was, therefore, a frequently heard cry in the 1890s. This was accompanied by a demand for "scientific medicine" to replace the rather haphazard "art." "In our efforts to maintain the dignity and protect the honor of our noble profession, we should see to it that none but men and women who have an interest in scientific medicine shall ever become a member of this or any county medical society," urged one important contemporary reformer to his local society.[26] In a society that was beginning to view technology and science as a new religion, few could argue against a purge of the "non-scientific" practitioners.

It is clear that the reform of medical education was almost a passion or a crusade. Despite the large costs of instituting laboratory procedures, clinical training programs, and other reforms during the 1890s, the laboratory, the hospital, and the university began, in a few instances, to replace the didactic lecture, the amphitheatre, and the independent medical school. In August of 1905, shortly after the AMA established its influential Council on Medical Education, *JAMA* presented a summary of the major objectives of reformers. The *Journal* maintained that the minimum requirement for admission should be "a first class high school education" and part or all of a regular college course. In the medical school itself, the demands centered around drastically revamping the didactic lecture courses that characterized the teaching method of many schools. Therefore, in the teaching of the "fundamental branches" of anatomy, physiology, physiologic chemistry, bacteriology, pathology, and pharmacology it was necessary to have "suitable, well-equipped" laboratories. All these changes required the expenditure of vast sums of money, as the *Journal* recognized. There needed to be "money for permanent buildings and equipment, and for annual appropriations for salaries and current expenses." The student's fees could no longer provide the money to cover these expenses. *JAMA* concluded, therefore, that "endowments and university connections are necessary."[27]

Both sources of funding were ardently pursued. The larger, predominantly eastern universities were able to tap the resources of industrial philanthropists. The plea for funds echoed throughout the society. One popular magazine editorialized that increased endowments were necessary to solve the financial crisis of many medical schools and the general crisis in medicine:

> We have too many doctors . . . and many of them are not well trained. Where the states cannot or will not equip [medical schools] and maintain them on the proper level of efficiency, private benefactors must. A million dollars given to such a school does more direct service to mankind, perhaps, than ten times as much money given to any other branch of education.[28]

A serious problem was associated with dependence of the medical school on philanthropy. Donation of money for medical education was a rare event. In fact, by the turn of the century there was a total of only $1,000,000 in endowments for all medical education. *JAMA* noted that "endowments to medical colleges [were] in the past among the rarest events in this country, not half a dozen institutions have received any considerable sums, and very few anything at all."[29]

Since private benefactors could not be depended upon to provide the necessary funds for very many schools, reformers turned to the state for the financing of medical education in areas outside the Northeast.[30] The focus of the reform movement in the southern, midwestern, and western states became the consolidation of all medical education into one state university medical school.[31]

The justification for having only one medical college in many of the less affluent states went beyond merely the practical "limited resources" issue that was so heavily touted in the editorial pages of *JAMA*. It was also justified on the grounds that fewer medical students would be produced. H. S. Pritchett, the president of the Carnegie Foundation, said in 1914 that "there is no justification for a second school of medicine in Indiana. One moderate-sized medical school, conducted along the right lines, can supply more physicians than the State of Indiana can possibly absorb."[32]

It is significant that most of the concern about the social status of medical practitioners and the desire to limit their number in the profession was voiced by *JAMA* and a few other eastern medical journals. One doctor explained medicine's lack of influence in the general community. He complained that "the truth is patent that very many of its members are persons of inferior ability, questionable character and coarse and common fiber."[33] He was dismayed not only by their incompetence but also by their "commonness." "Proprietary schools," private medical colleges that charged fees and whose professors made an indirect profit on their business, were major producers of this "common fiber" and were criticized by reformers on a wide variety of grounds. *JAMA* and others charged that they did not have the facilities for a superior education, that they were "commercialistic" rather than educational in their primary focus, and that they were lax in their standards. But equally disturbing to the critics was the fact that these schools trained representatives of the poor and the working class to be physicians. These institutions were, in short, encouraging the very kind and class of people the "profession" was trying to keep out. In his presidential address to the *AMA*, Dr. Billings talked with disdain of "these sundown institutions" that were organized for evening instruction and thus "enable the clerk, the streetcar conductor, the janitor and others employed during the day to earn a degree."[34] The AMA and others advocated the incorporation of medical schools into the university system not only to improve the quality of the physician's education but also to increase the doctor's social status. Dr. William Welch of Johns

Hopkins wrote in 1906: "The social position of the medical man and his influence on the community depend to a considerable extent upon his preliminary education and general culture."[35]

The AMA sought to reform medical education not only to create a class of "respectable" professionals but also to decrease the actual number of doctors so that the crucial overcrowding issue could be solved.[36] An editorial in *JAMA* was provokingly entitled, "Too Few Physicians? Hardly!" It tied the "excessive" number of medical schools to the overproduction of doctors. The *Journal* argued that if there were a drop in "the number of medical colleges by one half it would be a matter for serious regret."[37]

All this activity and rhetoric began to have the desired effects *before* the Flexner Report came out. The number of medical schools and students started dropping significantly in 1906 and continued at about the same pace before and after 1910, the year of the report's publication. In 1904, the peak year, there were 166 medical colleges in the United States. From 1905 to 1907 the number fluctuated between 160 and 161. By the time of the Flexner Report in 1910, the number had dropped to 133. This is not meant to imply that the Flexner Report was not important in several crucial respects. But what this evidence does indicate very strongly is that it was the AMA itself that played a large role in the "reform" of medical education and put the medical profession on the road to its present-day elitist, financially remunerative position.

The elimination of medical schools and lowering the number of physicians could be expected to affect different groups unevenly. *JAMA,* for instance, made it clear that there was "little reason to fear any undesirable falling off in the supply of undergraduates in the really high class institutions of the country."[38] Those would be mostly rich students in predominantly eastern universities. Who would suffer? One group that would be very hard hit by a standardized education supervised by the AMA were the non-regular colleges and physicians. The drop in attendance at these schools would be rather dramatic. The attendance at "regular" medical colleges grew until 1905 and then declined rather steadily. The number of students in homeopathic schools declined from 1900. The attendance at eclectic schools declined from a high of 1,014 in 1904 to 208 in 1912, and the physiomedical and nondescript schools were wiped out by 1912.[39]

Another group that was severely affected by this consolidation campaign was women physicians. The position of women in medicine, always weak, did not appear to be deteriorating prior to 1909. Although the number of medical colleges exclusively for women had decreased markedly, the percentage of women doctors and women graduates from medical colleges held steady. "From 1880 until 1904 . . . 4.3 percent [of M.D. degrees] were given to women," the *Women's Medical Journal* noted. "Yet in 1909," it continued approvingly, "the proportion of women graduates almost reached the high-water mark of five years ago, being 4.3 percent."[40] But this optimistic assessment was to be short-lived. By 1912 the percentage of women graduates had declined to 3.2 percent, as had the total number of women students.[41]

The decrease in the number of doctors, and the consolidation of medical schools were but one part of the changes occurring in medicine and medical education. For consolidation meant not only bigger and fewer medical schools but also the increasing takeover of hospitals and dispensaries by those medical schools that survived. In fact, the hospital was viewed as so necessary to a well-functioning medical school that *JAMA* editorialized in 1900 that "to a large extent the hospital, with [all its facilities], is the medical school."[42] By 1908 some noted that "the improvement of medical education [was and would be] closely allied with hospital growth" and use.[43] As early as 1900, ten years before the Flexner Report was to make the same observation, *JAMA* pointed to the need for a hospital completely controlled and managed by the university medical school. "It does not suffice," said the *Journal's* editor, "that this [medical school] hospital is adjacent to the college; it must be under the full and unrestricted management of the college, as far as the medical work is concerned."[44]

While certain medical schools were wealthy enough to build, equip, and staff their own hospitals, the vast majority of existing schools could not afford financially to do this. They had to find a hospital that would not only serve the medical school but also submit to its control. Numerous physicians acknowledged that a "primary" function of a hospital was to teach future physicians, but few could suggest how to get the hospital management to relinquish its control and hand it over to the medical school. In the early 1900s the hospitals were much more firmly established financially than were the numerous medical schools, and such an abrogation of control by hospital management could not be generally expected. Except for a few of the wealthier schools, such as Columbia, Harvard, and Johns Hopkins, the medical school had little it could offer the hospital other than personnel. The hospital, on the other hand, usually had a relatively stable source of income and, in the case of the charity hospital, an endowment. While the hospital management at the turn of the century was willing to take the cheap labor (the fourth-year student and intern) produced by the medical schools, they were less willing to give up political control over their institutions.

Exactly what kind of hospitals should be used for teaching purposes became a major question. As the impracticability of building their own hospitals became obvious to the medical schools, many suggested using public hospitals for teaching "because in most of [the private hospitals] the number of free or charity beds is . . . limited, and the private or pay patients are usually not at the disposal of the staff for teaching purposes to classes of medical students."[45] Even the representatives of medical schools that owned and controlled their own hospitals fostered the idea that the public hospital was the proper teaching facility for others.[46]

But the problem of gaining control of a public hospital was immense, and it was in this debate that a central theme of Progressive Era medical education reform is clearly seen. The consolidation of the public hospital and the medical school entailed taking these hospitals out of the "dirty politics" of government and placing them within the realm of "clean control" by the reforming medical school-university complexes.

While some saw the medical school as the vehicle by which the "dirty city politics" that interfered with the functioning of these institutions could be alleviated, others proposed alternative measures for removing the hospitals from popular control. Dr. Rupert Norton, assistant superintendent of Johns Hopkins Hospital, suggested that mayors should appoint a board of trustees, relatively independent of the vicissitudes of city politics and chosen "from the leading citizens, men who have shown their ability in the handling of big business organizations. . . . In this way the good government of the institution can be assured." Not only were the boards removed "from all evil political influences," but, furthermore they would select a superintendent whose "term should last indefinitely, under good behavior." In addition, in Norton's scheme, the superintendent, would "be left the real administration" and the board of trustees was to "serve in an advisory capacity" only.[47]

It is important to remember that the reform movement in medical education occurred at a time when the political machinery of the eastern cities was becoming more responsive to their increasingly immigrant constituencies. Insulating the hospitals and the profession from the "politics" of government meant that the rising elite of the medical profession could maintain control over the new, evolving medical system, even if local governments were no longer in their hands.

The foregoing has attempted to put the medical reform movement in perspective. We have tried to indicate that the impetus for medical education reform came from within the profession itself. Furthermore, substantial results were achieved *prior* to the issuance of the Flexner Report, and, in fact, the pace and rate of consolidation and elimination of medical colleges was as rapid *before* the report as after.

This is not to say, however, that Flexner's efforts were not important. It is clear that the Flexner Report strengthened the AMA's hand in the nation as a whole, for it was able to motivate an "independent educational agency such as the Carnegie Foundation" to substantiate and publicize the conditions and alternatives that the predominantly eastern, university-based, organized part of the profession wanted changed and adopted.[48] In addition, grants of vast sums of money were offered by the foundations to medical schools if their reforms followed Flexner's recomendations.[49]

Abraham Flexner himself clearly saw the need for reform in medical education and the increase in state powers to accomplish such upgrading as part of a larger movement in society. In an extremely significant article, he noted that in the simple, agrarian society of the early republic a small government was all that was necessary. But tremendous scientific advances had changed all that: "In order to avoid the dangers, in order to realize for the general welfare the largest possible measure of the potential benefits involved in scientific progress, the Government has had to enlarge its range of activity and interest." It was precisely "these general considerations which touch our entire national development" that made regulation of medical education a necessity.[50]

The Flexner Report also elicited a strong, if disunited, opposition to the vast changes it proposed for medicine and medical education. Alternative practitioners—blacks, women, and even a number of highly respected regular journals—opposed various aspects of the report. One journal attacked a fundamental basis of the report, that there were too many doctors. The *Alienist and Neurologist* complained that, in fact, there were not enough:

> When the public shall come to rightly realize the great need of medical emergency aid . . . now unprovided it will turn attention to systematic medical provision now ignorantly neglected and the recent senseless cry of "too many doctors" will cease to be heard in the land."[51]

Similarly, critics attacked the Flexner Report's stress on the need to eliminate the smaller medical colleges. "Carnegie 'and his men' and Rockefeller had better have endowed some of them," suggested one journal angrily. "Better lend strength to the weak than double the strength of the already strong."[52] A calmer, less radical statement of the same general viewpoint was made by *American Medicine.* It suggested that "the day of the small, comparatively inconsequential medical college is by no means passed."[53] Even *Popular Science Magazine* entered the fray, arguing that it would be better for the states to support "good schools [rather] than . . . suppressing those that are poor."[54]

Finally, opponents of the Flexner Report stressed the undemocratic and autocratic future that awaited the medical profession if it followed its present course. A thoughtful statement of this point of view was presented by the *New York State Journal of Medicine.* If, this journal asserted, it was unwise for the state to tell free and independent universities what to do, "What shall we say concerning a foundation [i.e., the Carnegie Foundation], itself the creature of the state which arrogates to itself powers not possessed by the state?" It continued by suggesting that such a situation was extremely dangerous. "An oligarchy within a republic is an anomaly. It is not the less anamalous because its intentions are good if its methods are such as to threaten the freedom of educational institutions."[55] Nor was this development seen as occurring in a vacuum. "Trade and commerce have for years been suffering from the dictation of powerful interests which have well nigh outgrown control both of courts and legislatures." Such a situation was clearly at hand in medical education as well. The *Journal* warned that the "mere possession or access to great wealth [should not] be the means of engrafting in our midst a sort of supreme educational council, self-perpetuating, responsible to no one—in fact, an educational oligarchy with the vast inertia of an immense fortune behind it."[56]

The reformers' actions and programs during the Progressive Era were in some senses progressive and necessary. The educational level of the average practitioner and his manner of care delivery were often limited. The private practitioner clung to an individualistic, small, isolated, competitive model. The AMA reformers thus sought to organize and professionalize doctors so that they might be "modern" practitioners.

While the AMA no doubt exaggerated the defects of the proprietary medical schools, for instance, there is no doubt that medical education needed reform. They did need labs and more individualized work. They did need clinical experience and observations. All this necessitated large sums of money, large schools, etc., which most of the proprietary schools could not afford to provide.

But it is equally important to understand that the way these changes and developments were accomplished was not necessary or the best. Furthermore, the rationale for centralization and bureaucratization was often confused. On the one hand, physicians thought like the class-conscious industrialists and acted to rationalize and modernize medicine. On the other hand, however, the AMA reformers depended on individual general practitioners for its collective clout and power. These physicians (along with the reformers) complained about their relative status and income and represented, collectively, a strong special interest group. They had neither the broad, national, progressive vision nor the class-conscious sophistication of their reform leaders. The result of the interaction of these two groups was change. But the reform was conservative in both intent and result. It was conservative not only in the sense that it concentrated power in the hands of a small elite but also in the sense that for the next half-century it protected the special self-interests of the practitioners. That is to say, the reforms centralized, bureaucratized, modernized, and expanded medicine and medical education in the interests of the physicians' own professional needs and to the exclusion of the needs of the public.

Notes

1. Elton Rayack, *Professional Power and American Medicine* (Cleveland: World Publishing, 1967), p. 37; see also Rosemary Stevens, *American Medicine and the Public Interest* (New Haven: Yale University Press, 1971), which is an important contribution to the literature.

2. Abraham Flexner, *Medical Education in the United States and Canada,* Carnegie Foundation, Bulletin No. 4. (New York, 1910).

3. See Richard Hofstadter, *The Age of Reform* (New York: Vintage Books, 1960), chap. 4, especially pp. 148-64, for his discussion of the responses of the urban middle classes to the growth of big business. Our interpretation differs substantially from Hofstadter's on the origins and nature of progressivism as a whole. For different views, see Howard Berliner, "A Larger Perspective on the Flexner Report," *International Journal of Health Services Research* 5 (1975): 573-92; and E. Richard Brown, *Rockefeller Medicine Men: Medicine and Capitalism in The Progressive Era* (Berkeley: University of California Press, 1979). Samuel Hays, *Conservation and the Gospel of Efficiency* (Cambridge: Harvard University Press, 1959), p. 3; James Weinstein, *The Corporate Ideal in the Liberal State* (Boston: Beacon Press, 1968), and Gabriel Kolko, *The Triumph of Conservatism* (New York: Free Press of Glencoe, 1963) for the business influence on reform.

4. Hays, p. 5.

5. J. M. Taylor, "Cooperation in Medicine," *Journal of the American Medical Association (JAMA)* 60 (7 June 1913): 1810.

6. "Our Prospects as a Profession," *JAMA* 31 (15 October 1898): 932.

7. W. S. Foster, "A Few Suggestions," *Pittsburgh Medical Review* 10 (June 1896): 176.

8. "The Social Training of the Physician," *JAMA* 44 (17 June 1905): 1933.

9. C. H. Reed, "Why is the Profession Poor in Purse? And How to Remedy It," *JAMA* 32 (6 May 1898): 975.

10. G. F. Shears, "Making a Choice," *Cosmopolitan* 34 (April 1903): 654.

11. "The Economics of Medicine," *New York State Journal of Medicine (NYSJ of M)* 9 (December 1909): 481.

12. "The Physician's Income," *Medical Record* 69 (17 February 1906): 264.

13. "Causes of the Decline of Physician's Incomes," *Medical News* 71 (23 October 1897): 534. For other discussion of the poor income of doctors, see also J. W. Harrington, "Physician," *Munsey* 25 (July 1901): 589; N. G. Price, "Reflections on the Financial Status of Doctors," *New York Medical Journal (NYMJ)* 80 (30 July 1898): 212; T. F. Reilly, "Medical Economics," *NYMJ* 96 (26 October, 1912): 843-47; B. Herman, "The Economic Difficulties of the G. P.," *American Medicine* 8 (May 1913), 298.

14. See e.g. C. N. Branin to ed., *JAMA* 55 (6 August 1910), 520.

15. R. A. Henderson, "The Division of Professional Fees," *American Medicine* 6 (November 1911): 577.

16. T. J. Happel, "Quo Vadis," *JAMA* 32 (11 February 1899): 273.

17. C. L. Girard, "A Comparison of the Old-time and Modern Physician," *Journal of Michigan Medical Society* 6 (March 1907): 107.

18. W. F. Campbell, "Economic Factors in the Doctor's Future," *Long Island Journal of Medicine* 7 (March 1913): 140.

19. "Distribution of Physicians," *JAMA* 37 (26 October 1901): 1,119; see also C. H. Reed, "Why is the Profession Poor in Purse?" *JAMA* 32 (6 May 1899): 976; and G. H. Rohe, "Proportion of Physicians to Population," *JAMA* 30 (12 February 1898): 386-87.

20. "Oversupply of Medical Graduates," *JAMA* 37 (27 July 1901): 270.

21. For other statements on overproduction, see also F. Billings, "Medical Education," *Science* 17 (May 1903): 771 (wants 2,500 grads and a maximum of 35 medical schools); Ibid., p. 762 ("There are evils which menace, chief of which still are too many medical schools, too many students. . . ."); "The Consolidation of Medical Colleges," *Illinois Medical Journal* 16 (August 1909): 206-07 (asserts that Illinois had too many schools); G. V. N. Dearborn, "How Can Standards of the Medical Profession be Raised," *American Medicine* 5 (11 April 1903): 588 (if reduced, "the graduate output for a few years the public would not suffer, while present practitioners would considerably benefit both in income and in experience"); "Too few physicians? Hardly!" *JAMA* 44 (27 May 1905): 1689.

22. T. L. Hatch, "Whither Are We Tending," *JAMA* 32 (7 January 1899): 39-40.

23. S. E. Chaillé, "The Practice of Medicine as a Money Making Occupation," *New Orleans Medical and Surgical Journal* 49 (May 1897): 608.

24. C. L. Girard, "A Comparison," *Mich. Med. Soc.* (1 April 1911): 973; I. W. Voorhees, "Economics of Medicine," *American Medicine* 8 (February 1913), 86.

25. "Medical Education and Colleges," *JAMA* 24 (1895): 66.

26. W. H. Welch, "Medical Advancement," *American Medicine* 6 (25 October 1903): 675.

27. "The Influence of the Private Practitioner in Medical Education," *JAMA* 45 (19 August 1905): 538-89; for similar views, see also the following: A. D. Bevan, "Medical Education in the United States - The Need of a Uniform Standard," *JAMA* 51 (15 August 1908): 566; H. J. Whitacre, "Medical Education," *Cincinnati Lancet-Clinical* 50 (7 February 1903):

135-48; A. L. Benedict and J. Madden,"Medical Education and the Education of Medical Men," *Review of Reviews* 12 (November 1895): 582-83; "Council on Medical Education of the American Medical Association," (1st Annual Conference Proceedings), *JAMA* 44 (6 May 1905): 1,470-75. On improving and professionalizing teaching, see, for example, "American Academy of Medicine," *JAMA* 53 (3 July 1909): 70; "The University Medical School," *JAMA* 39 (8 October 1902): 989. For improvement of laboratory instruction, see H. P. Bowditch, "Reform in Medical Education," *Science* 8 (30 December 1898), 922; H. P. Bowditch, "Medical School of the Future in the United States," *Science* 11 (4 May 1900): 695; C. W. Eliot, "Future of Medicine," *Science* 24 (12 October 1906).

28. "Do You Know," *World's Work* 22 (June 1911): 14, 441.

29. "Medical College Endowments," *JAMA* 35 (24 November 1900): 1,353; see also "Dr. Senn's Gift," *JAMA* 35 (10 November 1900): 1,217; "The Presidential Address," *JAMA* 34 (9 June 1900): 1,492; Hurd, "Duty of Medical Education,"*Science* 9 (17 July 1903): 72.

30. See "States and Municipalities and Medical Education," *JAMA* 51 (15 August 1908): 606.

31. "Medical Education in Alabama," *JAMA* 59 (1 October 1912); see "State Support of Medical Education,"*JAMA* 57 (5 August 1911): 487, in which the *Journal* of the AMA notes that "slowly but surely colleges . . . are either obtaining connections with privately endowed universities or are giving way to the state-supported university medical school"; also "Hospital and Clinical Work," *JAMA* 41 (15 August 1903): 429.

32. H. S. Pritchett, "The Medical School and the State," *JAMA* 63 (22 August 1914): 650.

33. I. C. Philbrick, "Medical Colleges and Professional Standards," *JAMA* 36 (15 June 1910): 1700.

34. F. Billings, "Medical Education," *Science* 17 (May 1903): 763.

35. W. H. Welch, "Unity," *Science* 24 (12 October 1906): 458.

36. F. Billings, "Medical Education," *Science* 17 (May 1903): 763-64; J. H. Musser, "Presidential Address," *JAMA* 42 (11 June 1904): 1,538.

37. "Too Few Physicians? Hardly!" *JAMA* 42 (27 May 1905): 1,989; I. C. Philbrick, "Medical Colleges," *JAMA* 36 (15 June 1901): 1,700; N. G. Price, "Reflections on the Financial Status of the Medical Career," *NYMJ* 80 (30 July 1904): 214; D. S. Jordan, "American Medical Schools," *BAAM* 9 (February 1908): 29-30.

38. "Too Few Physicians? Hardly!" *JAMA* 44 (27 May 1905): 1,689.

39. "Medical Education in U.S.," *JAMA* 59 (24 August 1912): 650 Similarly for medical schools: regular medical colleges decreased in number from 131 in 1907, to 123 in 1908, to 117 in 1909, to 111 in 1910, to 101 in 1911, to 100 in 1912. Homeopathic schools fell consistently from a high of 22 in 1900 to 10 in 1912. The eclectic schools fell from 19 in 1900 to 6 in 1912 and the physiomedicine and nondescript colleges were eliminated by 1911.

40. "Women Medical Students," *Women Medical Journal,* 19 (December 1909), 258.

41. "Medical Education in U.S.," *JAMA* 59 (24 August 1913): 650; C. C. Dana "The Doctor's Future," *NYMJ* 97 (4 January 1913): 3; see also

Ella Prentice Upham, "Women in Medicine," *North American Journal of Homeopathy* 56 (July 1908): 346-67, for figures on women doctors in America in 1900: 7,399 women doctors, of whom 1,067 were foreign born and 160 were blacks. For a paternalistic opposition to women in Medicine, see C. Cabot, "Women in Medicine," *JAMA* 65 (11 September 1915): 947-48; for defenses, see S. A. Knopf, "Professor Cabot and Women Physicians," *Lancet-Clinic* 113 (26 June 1915): 720; G. A. Walker, "The Women's Medical College of Pennsylvania," *Women's Medical Journal* 26 (February 1916): 44.

42. "Medical Schools and Hospitals," *JAMA* 35 (25 August 1900): 501. Although other early statements concerning the relationship between medical schools and hospitals were not as direct, many did suggest the widespread use of the hospital for teaching purposes; see "Charity Hospital and Resident Surgeon," *New Orleans Medical and Surgical Journal* 49 (January 1897): 413; W. Osler, "Natural Method of Teaching Medicine," *JAMA* 36 (15 June 1901): 1,672; "The Extramural Clinic" *JAMA* 39 (6 September 1902): 328-29; W. W. Keen, "Duties and Responsibilities of Trustees of Public Medical Institutions," *Science* 17 (22 May 1903): 806.

43. A. Post, "The Hospital in Relation to the Community," *Boston Medical and Surgical Journal* 158 (21 May 1908): 824.

44. "Medical and Hospital," *JAMA* 35 (25 August 1900): 501. For further evidence of the profession's desire for hospital-medical school consolidation, see B. Holmes, "The Hospital Problem," *JAMA* 47 (4 August 1906): 319; "Suggested Changes in Medical Education," *Boston Medical and Surgical Journal* 161 (8 July 1909); J. L. Heffron, "Hospitals and Their Relation to Medical Colleges and the Training of Interns," *JAMA* 62 (14 March 1914): 877; S. Flexner, "The Relation of Independent Institutions of Medicine to Medical Education," *Boston Medical and Surgical Journal* 160 (18 February 1909): 222-23; C. A. L. Reed, "The Modern Medical Colleges," *Lancet-Clinic* 102 (16 October 1909): 423.

45. C. R. Holmes, "Hospitals and Their Relation to Medical Schools," *American Medical Association Bulletin* 9 (1914): 299-313.

46. W. H. Welch, "Medicine and the University," *Science* 27 (3 January 1908): 16; see also "Medical Schools and Hospitals," *JAMA* 35 (25 August 1900): 501; J. P. Morgan, "Relation of the Clinical Professor to the Hospital, the Community, the Medical School, and the Profession," *Medical Record* 81 (8 June 1912): 1,081.

47. R. Norton, "Municipal Hospitals and their Relation to the Community," *JAMA* 61 (29 November 1913): 1,980.

48. See for this description, "Recent Progress in Medical Education in the U.S.," *JAMA* 58 (11 May 1912): 1,444; see also D. B. Munger, "Robert Brookings and the Flexner Report," *Journal of the History of Medicine* 23 (October 1968): 357, for the point that it was the Council on Medical Education itself that requested the Carnegie Foundation to do this report. J. Howland, "Medical Education," *Science* 32 (12 August 1910): 207.

49. See, for example, E. Richard Brown's article in this volume.

50. A. Flexner, "Medical Colleges," *World's Work* 21 (April 1911): 14,239.

51. "Not Enough Physicians," *Alienist and Neurologist* 32 (August 1911): 408. See also "Too Many Doctors? No! Not Enough," Ibid., February 1911, p. 203: "The people need medical advice and often treatment earlier and oftener than they seek it."

52. "Destruction of Independent Medical Schools," *Alienist and Neurologist* 32 (November 1911): 693.

53. "Medical Education," *American Medicine* 5 (September 1910): 442.

54. "Medical Education in the U.S.," *Popular Science* 77 (July 1910): 101; see also F. M. Gould, "A Vocation or Avocation?" *American Journal of Clinical Medicine* 15 (January 1908): 17: support for small versus large colleges ("Success, ambition, politics, greed, conservatism, the dirty kind—are more certain to rule the minds and kill the hearts of the men in control of the huge institutions than those of the small ones").

55. "The Carnegie Foundation," *NYSJM* 10 (November 1910): 483.

56. Ibid., p. 484; see also Edward W. Watson, "Medical Socialism," *Medical Notes and Queries* (Pa.) 5 (June 1910): 124-25: "In short, this new institute, these few men, are already assuming the right to manage the profession, to overthrow its traditions, and to rebuild it to Socialistic (!) lines." Chancellor MacCracken of New York University, quoted in W. G. Tucker, "Address," *Science* 26 (8 November 1907): 615.

11 The Search for the Hospital Yardstick: Nursing and the Rationalization of Hospital Work

Skyrocketing costs and seemingly irrational, unbusinesslike procedures have been the major problems ascribed to health care institutions in the 1970s. As concern over these issues has grown, the mantle of service and charity, which for so long has covered hospitals and other health care facilities, has slowly been removed. No longer minor parts of the economy, the hospitals have become business behemoths. They are now expected to run according to capitalist logic as much as any automobile plant or department store.

Because hospitals are labor intensive, much of the concern has focused on ways to curb labor costs and to rationalize the work process.[1] The nurses, because they are the largest group within the hospital work force, have come under particular attention. Attempts to manage and control the nurses are not new, however; only the forms it takes are different. This article will explore the relationship between hospitals and nursing by examining the managerial reforms for control over the work force and the role that nurses and other direct patient care workers played in bringing about these changes from the last

This paper was originally presented as part of a panel on "Management Reform and Women's Work" at the American Historical Association convention in 1976. Support from the Milbank Memorial Fund made the research possible. The author wishes to thank the following for their comments on earlier drafts: Susan Porter Benson, Rosalyn Feldberg, Maurine Greenwald, Diana Long Hall, Lise Vogel, Tim Sieber, David Rosner, Harry Marks, David Montgomery, Sam Bass Warner, Jr., the Work Relations Group.

quarter of the nineteenth century to the early 1950s. This approach suggests that the labor process in hospitals was shaped by the need of organized nursing to establish its professional status and by the concern of the hospitals to have a loyal work force. I will be examining general tendencies in this process, aware that hospitals are notoriously idiosyncratic facilities where policies can vary between floors, departments, and institutions.

When the editor of the journal *Hospital Management* was searching for an appropriate date for the first annual National Hospital Day in 1921, he settled on May 12—neither the anniversary of a medical breakthrough, nor the founding date of a great hospital, but the birthday of Florence Nightingale.[2] This symbolic gesture suggests both how closely the histories of hospitals and nursing are tied and how much hospital managements wanted to share in the charitable and saintly image of "the lady with the lamp." But in 1921 hospitals were no longer just charitable institutions and 75 percent of the "ladies with the lamps" were not working in them.[3]

Hospitals, of course, have always had someone performing some kind of nursing function. Up until the last quarter of the nineteenth century it was frequently the patients, expected to care for one another when they were ambulatory. There were usually some women employed as nurses but they were mostly unskilled and provided low level domestic functions. Many were on loan from the adjoining almshouses, although others worked in the hospitals permanently and gained a modicum of skills.[4] An occasional middle or upper class "lady" might be trained on the job as head nurse or matron.

The important change in the hospital's nursing work force began in 1873 when the first nurses' training schools were established. Some of the early schools were independent institutions with their own boards, but by the 1880s most schools were organized and controlled by the hospitals, who used the students as a source of non-wage labor. Nursing students were given only small allowances and, along with untrained attendants, became the major employees of most hospitals until the 1930s.

The growth of the hospitals was in part tied to the growth in nursing schools. In 1873, when the first nursing schools were founded, there were 178 hospitals in the United States. By 1923 there were 6,830 hospitals (an increase of over 3,700 percent), and every fourth one included a nursing school. By 1941 the number of hospitals had dropped by 7 percent because of the Depression, but the number of beds had increased by 75 percent.[5]

The two-class health delivery pattern of the late nineteenth and early twentieth centuries meant that upper-class and upper-middle class patients retained private duty nurses in their homes, or occasionally in hospitals. The poor and working class, especially if they were charity cases, relied on the hospitals and dispensaries. By the 1920s private-duty home care was becoming less common, the hospitals were being used more by all classes, while the two classes of care continued within and between institutions.[6]

The change in the role of hospitals beginning in the Progressive Era was not due to medical science and specialization alone, but also to urbanization, competition for patients between physicians, nurses, and hospitals, and a fiscal crisis within the hospitals resulting in declines in their philanthropic and public charity incomes.[7] Particularly in voluntaries and proprietaries, administrators and trustees had to devise schemes to bring in paying customers as a legitimate way to ease their financial difficulties. They had to convince the general populace that the hospitals were no longer just places where the poor were left to die.[8] In 1908 the superintendent of St. Luke's Hospital in Chicago bluntly declared at an American Hospital Association convention:

> If we can make our hospitals sufficiently attractive to induce patients to remain during convalescence, to come for diagnosis instead of going to hotels and visiting the doctor at his office and to come in for treatment of more or less chronic forms of disease, we will not only increase the number of possible patrons, but the prolonged stay will mean added work and further, the average profit per patient will be greater.[9]

To the administrators what was being created was both a "workshop for physicians" and a "modern hospital hotel."[10]

Yet the administrators and trustees had an ambivalence about these changes; they shared a sense of hope and a vision of their institutions as scientific centers and efficient businesses, as well as a real uncertainty about giving up their traditions of charity and paternalism.[11] However slowly, hospital care was becoming a commodity, not a charity. Patient payments were becoming the hospitals' most important income source.[12] As health care in the hospitals began to be sold to an increasingly higher class of patients, the administrators and trustees became more and more concerned with their "sales-force." Hospital care may have become a commodity, but it was still one being produced, despite the rhetoric, in a workshop by a largely undifferentiated work force. Unlike commodity producers, however, hospital administrators and trustees did not understand how to determine their own costs, labor or otherwise, lacked any real concept of how to measure productivity, and even questioned if it should be measured at all.

But they were caught up in the early twentieth century rhetoric and concern for efficiency. Many of the businessmen on the boards of trustees, although often aware that the hospital and their own enterprises were quite different, nevertheless felt that an efficient operation, from increasing the number of pay patients to improved nursing service, was part of the hospital's moral obligation to the community. In 1914, appropriately, they invited Frank Gilbreth, one of the fathers of scientific management, to speak at the hospital convention. Gilbreth was highly critical of the hospitals' lack of standardization and haphazard organization of work. The commentator on his paper gave lipservice agreement to his ideas. However, the journal *Modern Hospital* reflected the more widespread view when it reprinted his speech, not the commentary, and editorialized that the "dollar yardstick" alone could not be used to measure the hospital's worth.[13]

But the administrators and trustees did believe they needed a new yardstick to measure their employees' worth. As one administrator ruefully commented, "a $15-a-week clerk may have it in her power to alienate a $50,000-a-year endowment," or to drive patients away.[14] Thus, after financing, the most crucial problem, as the administrators perceived it, was the disciplining of their work force.[15]

Nineteenth- and early twentieth-century hospital management practices reflected the charity outlook, the unskilled and menial nature of most of the work, and the religious and military origins of hospitals and nursing. Under the rubric that the hospital was a family, the male superintendent (if there was one) or the chief surgeon was regarded as the father, the nursing school superintendent or matron was the mother, and the workers, nursing students, and patients were the children.[16] Both patients and workers were seen as recipients of the institution's charity. Workers were disciplined, like children, through the hospital's control over their daily lives: their food, housing, clothing, sexual activities, even the hours they slept. Rigid lines of authority were reinforced through separate housing, entrances, and dining facilities.

Women's boards often served as the workers' supervisors, trying to enforce middle-class standards of domestic amenities and measuring work success as if it were domestic service in their homes.[17] Thus appearances, docility, sobriety, cleanliness and speed, measured by the window shades aligned in a ward or the coverlets on the patients' beds pulled tight by 8 a.m., were all signs of proper worker behavior. But hospital managements fully expected their employees, whom they saw as morally flawed, to steal, to cheat the institution at every turn, and to quit with regularity.[18] Despite the paternalism, as Charles Rosenberg has argued, the hospitals frequently had a culture and life of their own over which the administrators, trustees, and visiting committees had very little control.[19]

Nursing students were also subject to this paternalism. Nursing superintendents were responsible for the education of the students, what little of it there was, but mainly for the actual staffing of the hospitals with these students. As would be employees, students were replaced whenever dropouts occurred. There was little concern for admission standards other than health and strength. Discipline, order, cleanliness, and respectability were all to be the hallmarks of this new creation—the hospital-trained nurse. Character, tact, and obedience, as well as antiseptic and aspetic techniques, were the new nurse's major skills.

Nursing schools ran under a rigid disciplinary model that was supposed to teach "idealism" and "implicit, unquestioning obedience" to a stunted matriarchy in which power only moved downward from the superintendent to the lowliest, newly arrived probationer.[20] Tasks were learned through constant repetition and adherence to each hospital's "one right way," not the "one best way," of performance. A nurse wrote of her training school experience at the turn of the century: "Good care of patients . . . is not made to depend on the individual nurse any more than is absolutely necessary. It is more a matter of a routine being established whose proper working will prevent mistakes on the part of a worker."[21]

Nurses, when they graduated, usually were not employed by hospitals because they were too expensive, too hard to discipline, and too willing to quit. Only those nurses with what was called "executive ability" might expect institutional appointments, and these positions were as nursing superintendents or head nurses, not as general staff nurses.[22] Most graduate nurses therefore became individual entrepreneurs in the uncertain private duty market, where they worked primarily for middle- and upper-class patients in their homes.[23] Those few who accompanied their patients into the hospitals were seen by hospital administrators and nursing matrons as almost dangerous interlopers whose independence might disturb family tranquility.[24]

In private duty the graduates competed for positions with the untrained, with nursing school dropouts, correspondence school, and short-course nurses. By the 1890s nurses in the major cities were complaining about overcrowding, limited training, overwork, and the way in which access to private duty was controlled by the hospitals and physicians running the major nursing registries.[25] The graduate nurse was caught in an ambiguous position. She was a "professional" worker who was expected to perform servant duties; an independent worker who was paid a standard wage and had a busy and slow season like a factory hand; and a skilled worker who was not given any financial incentive, training, or supervision to improve her skills.

When rank-and-file nurses articulated this situation as a severe problem, they were generally blamed by hospitals, physicians, and by many nursing leaders for their lack of character and concern for patients; their "inability" to choose the proper training school; for their refusal to organize under the leadership of nursing educators whose interests they might see as inimical to their own.[26] Revolt on the part of the nurses was primarily individual: refusing to work for physicians they disliked or distrusted, or to take certain types of difficult cases, gossiping about the hospitals, "floating" from city to city in search of work, or leaving nursing altogether.[27]

By the 1910s the nursing leadership (made up of nursing school superintendents and educators from the larger schools through the National League for Nursing Education and the American Nurses Association), saw that the solution to overcrowding and lack of training in nursing lay in fewer schools, higher admission standards, and less hospital control over the student's education. At the same time, hospital administrators began to realize that their patients were reluctant to accept lower-class workers or untrained students and were bringing more private duty nurses with them into the instututions. Administrators had to agree to some kind of upgrading or training to retain control over their work force. These concerns intensified between 1910 and World War II because of the workers' and nursing students' own response to their conditions.

Nursing leaders complained during the 1920s that women with the "right character" and "proper home training" were not applying to nursing school and that the public saw the school, with its rigidities, as "a sort of respectable reform school where its mental or disciplinary cases can be sent."[28] By the late 1910s and 1920s, as more occupations and white-collar positions were opened for the daughters of the middle class, nursing was attracting more working-class than middle-class women to its ranks.[29] May Ayres Burgess, the influential author of a 1928 study that was nursing's equivalent to medicine's Flexner Report in 1910, warned both nursing leaders and hospital administrators that the problem was class:

> These undereducated, unprepared women make trouble within the profession. Many of them are drawn from a social group which is not strictly professional in character. They are the ones who are talking trade unionism for nurses. It is natural that they should. Their fathers, brothers, and sweethearts are ardent members of trade unions. . . . Somehow these undereducated women, of inadequate social and academic background must be kept out of the profession. Fortunately, there is no longer any need for them.[30]

Her fears about unionism were based mainly on future possibilities, although there had been sporadic strikes and union organization among nursing students, nurses, and hospital workers since the 1890s.[31]

On the whole, nurses, nursing students, and other workers in hospitals relied upon subtler forms of revolt. Administrators complained that they refused to answer call buttons, to file reports, to clean up properly, to accept discipline, and would mix medications, complain to patients about the faults of the hospitals, and socialize with each other on hospital time.[32] What they did most visibly was quit. By the 1920s and 1930s hospitals began to realize, as had other industries, that the high turnover rates that they had accepted as inevitable were exceedingly expensive. Improved conditions appeared to be the only solution to the turnover crisis and a way to thwart trade union activity.[33]

The response of hospital administrators and nursing superintendents took several different forms. In general, they made attempts to transform the workers' character rather than to change the actual work process or the inequitable social hierarchy. As in other service industries where the workers' *behavior* is actually part of what is being sold, the administrators concentrated on changing the amenities and refurbishing their nineteenth-century paternalism in order to obtain a more loyal work force.[34]

Since nurses and workers were often housed in garrets in odd corners of the institutions, administrations began to build fancier nurses' homes, better dining rooms, etc., although the social distinctions between facilities for the different levels of workers were continued.[35] By the Depression the hospitals were moving away from providing full maintenance for all employees with the exception of the nurses. By the 1940s the trend had come full circle and administrators were counseled to "redefine the relationship of employees to the hospital. . . . Non-resident employees should consider the hospital their place of employment and not their home."[36]

Secondly, the appeals for loyalty and greater work effort were made in the language of "joint efficiency" and "mutual cooperation" rather than charitable duties.[37] Since little was done to relieve the drudgery or low pay of the work, in the mid-1920s hospital administrators began to discuss reliance upon a loyal cadre of workers. They later defined this as making it possible to have "the gradual shifting of external authority to internal authority, that is, to an increasing amount of self-control and self-direction."[38] Loyalty was to be obtained by proper training of workers and nursing students to their hierarchical position and to the service ethic of the hospital. The

213

concept of "our hospital" has a more honest ring than when such language becomes "our store" or "our company." Many workers and nurses did feel that way about the hospitals and did have a sense of pride and commitment to caring for patients and sharing the burden of their work. In case the workers did not already have such sentiments, a general service foreman in a San Francisco hospital pointed out "training will imbue them with this essential characteristic."[39] What was new in all of this was that the human relations and industrial psychology techniques of industry were being transplanted to the hospitals. Supervisors, for example, were told to learn about workers' families, to support employee efforts for hard work, and, above all, "to encourage the achievement of personnel stability through the development of personnel loyalty."[40] During the 1920s workers who did not wear uniforms were urged to accept them; administrators hoped this would be a way to promote discipline and instill institutional personalities.[41]

These methods, however, were not employed on a widescale basis, and instead many hospitals came to rely, as did other industries, upon a "flying squadron"—a small core of loyal workers who could be called upon to do a variety of jobs within the hospital.[42] But if the hospital gained this loyal core, it also gained a strong informal network of an "old guard," especially among the nurses. Made up primarily of older single women, these nurses lived together in the hospital residences for nurses and had connections to doctors and the boards of trustees that allowed them to subvert the hospitals' supposed command structures. *Modern Hospital* journal suggested that administrators fire such women when necessary, but such tactics were often unsuccessful when these women had cultivated such high-placed support.[43]

Hospitals were constantly searching for workers who could be relied upon to be loyal, self-motivating within set limits, imbued with the service ethic, willing to accept low wages and their place in a hierarchy, and yet able to transcend normal work loads when emergencies (defined by the administration) or shortages occurred. In the 1920s and 1930s, as medical and nursing practice became more technical and complex, they also began to need nurses who could provide more skilled work. Coupled with organized nursing's desire to upgrade the nurse's position, hospital administrators and nursing leaders together worked out a solution to both their dilemmas: They began to differentiate between the delivery of *nursing care* (which only a trained RN could provide) and the establishment of a *nursing service* (a team of nursing workers on different skill levels).

As early as 1909 the American Hospital Association had suggested the creation of trained subsidiary nursing workers, and physician committees were always suggesting that "sub-nurses" were really needed.[44] But as long as hospitals and most of the nursing superintendents were convinced that nursing students and untrained attendants were cheaper and more effective, the hospitals were unwilling to begin to think in terms of graded work and a trained assistants' staff. "It was an extraordinary thing," a national nursing report concluded in 1928, "but it seems to be a fact that hospitals regard the suggestion that they pay for their own nursing service as unreasonable . . . the student nurse is seen as an inalienable right."[45] Many nurses also feared that trained nursing assistants would unleash more legitimized lower-priced competition into the already overcrowded private duty market. But if these workers could be given different uniforms, be trained separately, do different work, come from a lower-class or lower-status ethnic group than nurses, as well as stay employed in the hospitals, their threat could be minimized.[46]

Thus, in every generation of nurses there were nursing leaders, many of whom were both nursing educators and hospital administrators, who increasingly saw nursing's future professional status as tied to a rationalized hospital nursing system with a complex division of labor.[47] It was primarily these women who convinced the hospitals both to upgrade the nurse and to subdivide her work because it would be cheaper for hospitals, would give them a disciplined work force through hierarchy and professionalism, and would improve the quality of care. At the turn of the century, they began by questioning the strict ward discipline, citing the fact that the absolute control of the physicians was "short-sighted policy from a business point of view."[48] They argued both that scientific management techniques were applicable to nursing work and that nurses were already unconsciously using them.

It was precisely a concern with detail, systemizing and proper organization that trained nursing brought to the hospitals. In practice this was usually translated into rigidity and mindless repetition of set patterns. But among nursing's more educated leadership, there was a real willingness to experiment with different forms of work organization and a belief that better training and planning could upgrade the nurse's status and dignity. Anne Goodrich, a nursing educator from Columbia and Yale universities, told the Harvard Medical Club in 1915, "No one is more concerned than a nurse in this standardization of hospitals."[49] Minnie Goodnow, another nursing superintendent and nursing historian, informed the annual hospital convention that nurses were training students "as Mr. Gilbreth does his bricklayers, and as all the efficiency engineers are doing in factories and business offices."[50] M. Adelaide Nutting, the nursing superintendent at Johns Hopkins and later the first full professor of nursing at Columbia, was also interested in the application of scientific management to institutional and home management. A founding member of the American Home Economics Association, she had contacted Lillian Gilbreth, a leading efficiency expert, to enlist her in studying household tasks.[51] The concern with scientific management in both industry and home was therefore transferred by the nurses into the hospitals. By the 1920s the National League for Nursing Education introduced some of the first time-and-motion studies of nursing work.[52]

The major catalyst for change, however, was the Depression, which created another financial crisis for the hospitals. Their income dropped precipitously when demand increased as patients, who could no longer afford either private nursing or physicians, flocked to what they still considered to be charity institutions.[53] Private duty nurses, for whom the Depression had begun in the mid-1920s, found themselves at the point of starvation. By 1932 the American Nurses Association had to send a letter to every hospital in the country urging them to accept graduate nurses on their staffs, to close their nursing schools, and to employ ward assistants.[54] Study after study began to appear in both the nursing and hospital management literature comparing student and graduate labor. The studies were attempts to convince hospitals and reluctant nursing superintendents that graduate nurses were more efficient workers, cheaper because of low wage demands, and easier to discipline both because of their professionalism and because they would be the hospitals' not the patients' employees.[55]

But hospitals were still reluctant to hire graduates as staff nurses. Many institutions did close their nursing schools and the number of schools dropped by 30 percent between 1929 and 1939.[56] But many hospitals substituted a variation on the private-duty system called group nursing. The graduate nurse became a hospital employee but was used only with groups of private patients in special rearranged rooms. This allowed the hospital to charge patients extra for this service rather than include it as part of routine hospital care.[57]

The nursing leaders had to convince both hospitals and nurses that the solution to everyone's problems was to have the graduate become a general duty worker in the hospital, not some modified private-duty nurse. They faced a reluctant rank and file who saw in hospital work a return to the drudgery, exploitation, and low status they associated with nursing school and institutional employment. Surveys of nursing registries in 1934 and again in 1937 concluded that nurses "are unwilling to accept prevailing conditions of employment for general staff nursing."[58]

The conditions in the hospitals included twelve- and fourteen-hour days on split shifts, excessively strenuous work, rotations from service to service, inadequate pay (often only room and board or a daily salary pro-rated on a monthly basis), and dismissals when the hospital census dropped. Above all, it meant that once in the hospital the nurse lost her one-to-one relationship with a patient and gained, in the language of the hospital, a "patient load."[59] Overcrowding of patients and understaffing of nurses were chronic dilemmas. For nurses, for whom the very definition of their work was service and comfort to individual patients, the work in hospitals was often an anathema. The nurses reported: "Floor duty in hospitals is too hard and often with not enough help, and one had no time to do the little things for patients that often mean much to add to their comfort and health."[60] But in the hospital the nurse did gain some promise of regular employment when economic conditions were improved. The incorporation of nurses into the hospital became common during the nursing shortages of World War II and in the early 1950s. Time-and-motion studies were used to create a nursing team that divided functions and then assigned them to different level workers, making the RN the foreman of the team.

In the words of contemporary critics of current nursing practices, nurses traded control over patient care for some control over other workers.[61]

It should be recalled that in 1914 the hospital administrators and trustees were uncertain about the feasibility of using Frank Gilbreth's yardstick. As late as their 1962 convention, they even showed a film, "Sam Sliderule Surveys the Hospital" which asserted that the efficiency studies of the industrial engineer were not necessarily applicable to the modern hospital.[62] But beginning in the 1920s and growing in the 1950s, nurses provided the hospitals with what they called a "nursing yardstick" by working with industrial engineers, including Lillian Gilbreth, the mother of scientific management, and by sponsoring during the early 1950s over thirty-four studies on nursing functions in seventeen states.[63] The authors of a major hospital engineering textbook in 1966 stated reluctantly: "It is difficult to escape the conclusion that the initiative for the adoption of industrial engineering concepts to hospital activities during the post war years came in large measure from nurses."[64]

But this ultimately proved to be a solution for the hospitals and not for the majority of nurses. As nursing functions were continually spun off, the nurse found herself increasingly task-oriented, tied to paperwork; the nursing station became further and further removed from direct patient care, and the nurse responsible for patients she often never saw or touched. Once incorporated into the administration of the hospital, many nurses quickly gained a stake in its smooth functioning. Advancement in nursing for a few consisted of climbing up the hospital hierarchical ladder, and meant implicit acceptance of the institution's terms. Yet because the hospital's idea of efficiency meant the use of as inexpensive a worker as possible, nurses found themselves (despite legal regulations to the contrary), often doing the same work as aides or licensed practical nurses and trying desperately to define and justify what the differences were between their skills.[65] Chronic understaffing meant nurses were shifted from floor to floor whenever administrators defined the need. As a result, nursing strikes and bargaining issues in the last thirty years have been primarily over staffing patterns and definitions of nursing functions.[66]

As hospitals emerged from their charity base in the twentieth century, they grew not so much into full-blown, rationalized, capitalist factories as into capitalist service institutions. As such, their nineteenth-century paternalism was reformed to meet twentieth-century conditions, rather than abandoned. Eric Perkins' view of southern planter-slave relations is equally relevant to hospitals. He points out that "paternalism was never 'pure' in the South because it had to constantly confront the infection of capitalist relations of production and the values associated with it, values measured not by duty or obligation, but by profit and loss."[67] In the hospitals profit and loss were measured less in cash terms and more by numbers of patients, expansion, prestigous research and education; but the same "infection" ran rampant. For the work force, the symptoms were low pay, poor working conditions, high turnover, and constant pressures to accept institutionally defined norms of proper character and service.

Scientific management was therefore more rhetoric than reality in the hospitals in the first half of this century. Nursing leaders, fueled by their need to find nurses a viable work place and to establish their professional role, saw scientific management concepts as meeting their needs and making their work easier. Nursing leadership has continued to see the creation of hierarchy and a caste system as a solution to nursing's professional difficulties. But as nursing leaders struggled to establish the scientific management of nursing work, they were constantly confronted by the objective difficulty of transforming service work into commodity production, the hospitals' unwillingness to use more skilled and expensive labor, and revolts from their own rank and file.

Recent works in nursing history suggest that sexism, male greed, and women's passivity explain nurses' subordination. But nurses must not be seen solely as victims or heroines in a male-dominated system. We must understand both why certain nursing leaders chose the direction they did and how and why their rank and file responded. The American Nurses Association bicentennial history book is entitled *One Strong Voice,* but even a beginning examination of nursing history suggests that there has always been a chorus.

Notes

1. The focus on labor costs has been, in part, because the other costs in the hospitals have been more protected. The use of third-party reimbursements to cover the costs of an additional piece of fancy technology or pay bank interest charges can be more hidden or justified than wage increases.

2. "First National Hospital Day May 12, Organized Effort to Educate Public as to Service of Institutions Begun by HOSPITAL MANAGEMENT, Every Hospital to Benefit," *Hospital Management* 11 (March 1921): 30-33; Malcolm T. MacEachern, "How are You Going to Celebrate National Hospital Day?" *Hospital Management (HM)* 31 (April 1931): 22-26.

3. May Ayres Burgess, *Nurses, Patients and Pocketbooks, Report of A Study of the Economics of Nursing Conducted by the Committee on the Grading of Nursing Schools* (New York, 1928), pp. 248-50.

4. Charles Rosenberg, "And Heal the Sick: The Hospital and the Patient in 19th Century America," *Journal of Social History* 10 (June 1977): 428-47.

5. U. S. Bureau of Census, *Historical Statistics of the United States from Colonial Times to 1957* (Washington, D.C., 1959), Series B 192-94, 235-36; Committee on Hospital Care, *Hospital Care in the United States* (Cambridge, Mass., 1947 and 1957), pp. 52-54.

6. David Rosner, "A Once Charitable Enterprise" (Ph.D. Diss., Harvard University, Dept. of History of Science, 1978); Morris Vogel, "Boston's Hospitals, 1880-1930, A Social History" (Ph.D. diss., University of Chicago, Dept. of History, 1974); Health Policy Advisory Center, *The American Health Empire: Power, Profits and Politics* (New York, 1970).

7. Rosemary Stevens, *American Medicine and the Public Interest* (New Haven, 1971); the analysis is based in part upon my examination of hospital management journals and texts beginning in the 1890s. See also David Rosner's article in this volume.

8. David Rosner has found that the Brooklyn hospitals began to aggressively advertise their "advantages" during the Progressive Era. In 1923 Somerville Hospital in Somerville, Massachusetts, sent an envelope home with all the school children of the city that informed their parents that: "Your little child might be the next one picked up from underneath a machine and rushed to Somerville Hospital for first aid and his little life saved—THE ONLY HOSPITAL in the city with its doors always open for such cases" (*30th Annual Report,* Somerville Hospital [Somerville, 1923], n.p).

9. Louis Curtis, "The Modern Hotel-Hospital," *National Hospital Record (NHR)* 11 (15 January 1908): 7.

10. Ibid.; George Rosen, "The Hospital: Historical Sociology of a Community Institution," *From Medical Police to Social Medicine* (New York, 1974), pp. 294-303; Del T. Sutton, "Three Years of Growth in the Hospital Field," *NHR* 3 (August 1900): 21-26; John A. Hornsby, "The Modern Hospital—A New Entity," *Modern Hospital (MH)* 1 (October 1913): 112-13; Frederick D. Keppel, "The Modern Hospital as a Health Factory," *MH* 7 (October 1916): 303-06.

11. See, for example, Charlotte Aikens, *Hospital Management* (Phila-
delphia, 1911); Frank Chapman, *Hospital Organization and Operation*
(New York, 1924); Ernest Codman, *A Study in Hospital Efficiency*
(Boston, n.d.); John Hornsby and Richard Schmidt, *The Modern Hospital*
(Philadelphia, 1913); Albert Ochsner and Meyer Strum, *The Organization,
Construction and Management of Hospitals* (Chicago, 1909).

12. C. Rufus Rorem, *The Crisis in Hospital Finance* (Chicago, 1932),
pp. 109-15.

13. Frank Gilbreth, "Scientific Management in the Hospital," *Transactions of the American Hospital Association (TAHA),* 16th Annual Convention (St. Paul, Minn., 1914), pp. 483-92; Dr. Anker, "Comments on
Gilbreth," Ibid., pp. 493-94; "The Dollar Yardstick," *MH* 3 (November
1914): 318.

14. "Friendliness in the Hospital," *MH* 12 (January 1919): 46.

15. "A Symposium on Hospital Discipline," *NHR* 7 (June 1905): 30-
35; John Hornsby, "Homes for Hospital Employees," *MH* 2 (June 1914):
365-66.

16. See, for example, Nina Dale, "The Hospital Family—Cooperation
in Domestic Management," *MH* 3 (September 1914): 187-89; Amy Beers,
"How Nurses May Contribute toward a Hospital's Success," *MH* 3 (November 1914), 302-04; Asa Bacon, "Nurses and Factory Labor," *MH* 8 (April
1917): 299; Charlotte Aikens, "Some Opportunities for Young Women
Outside the Nursing Field," *NHR* 11 (1 April 1908): 3-4; George H. M.
Rowe, "Observations on Hospital Organization," *NHR* 6 (December
1902): 3-10; this point is more fully developed in JoAnn Ashley, *Hospitals,
Paternalism and the Role of the Nurse* (New York, 1976).

17. Janet Wilson James, "Women and the Development of Health and
Welfare Services in Industrial America, 1870-1890," paper presented at the
Berkshire Conference on the History of Women, June 1976.

18. "Hospital Employees Welfare," *MH* 17 (September 1921): 214;
Temple Burling et al., *The Give and Take in Hospitals* (New York, 1956),
p. 61; Henry C. Wright, *Report of the Committee of Inquiry into the
Departments of Health, Charities, and Bellevue and Allied Hospitals in the
City of New York* (New York, 1913), pp. 77-78, 555, 596; Hornsby and
Schmidt, p. 66; "Discipline," *Trained Nurse and Hospital Review (TN &
HR)* 50 (February 1913): 101-02; for the similarity with domestic service,
see Lucy M. Salmon, *Domestic Service* (New York, 1897).

19. See note 4, above.

20. Isabel Hampton Robb, *Nursing Ethics* (Cleveland, 1901), p. 46;
similarly, see Charlotte Aikens, *Studies in Ethics for Nurses* (Philadelphia,
1916); Lavinia L. Dock, "The Relation of Training Schools to Hospitals,"
Nursing of the Sick 1893, reprint of the papers and discussions from the
International Congress of Charities, Correction, and Philanthropy, Chicago,
1893 (New York, 1949), p. 20.

21. "With Humanity Left Out" (Letter to the Editor from a nurse),
TN & HR 59 (November 1919): 706.

22. Nancy Tomes, "'Little World of Our Own': The Pennsylvania Hospital Training School for Nurses, 1895-1907," *Journal of the History of
Medicine and Allied Sciences,* forthcoming.

23. Susan Reverby, " 'Neither for the Drawing Room nor for the Kitchen,' Private Duty Nurses, 1873-1914," paper presented at the Organization of American Historians Convention, April 1978.

24. "The Special Nurse" (Letter to the Editor from "HBJ") *TN & HR* 54 (February 1915): 107; Hornsby and Schmidt, *passim;* Janet Geister, "Hearsay and Facts in Private Duty," *American Journal of Nursing (AJN)* 26 (July 1926): 80-93.

25. See note 23, above. See also Lavinia L. Dock, "Overcrowding in the Nursing Profession," *TN & HR* 22 (July 1898): 8-13; Anita Newcomb McGee, "The Growth of the Nursing Profession in the U.S.," *TN & HR* 24 (June 1900): 442-45; "Is the Profession becoming Overcrowded?" *AJN* 3 (April 1903): 513-15; "An Over-Supply of Nurses," *Pacific Coast Nursing Journal* 10 (January 1914): 3.

26. Between 1897 and 1903 a debate raged in the pages of the *Trained Nurse* on the type of nursing organization that should be formed in New York State, illustrating both the division between rank-and-file graduate nurses and their superintendents and the nature of the attacks on graduate nurses. See "To the Graduate Nurses of New York State" (Letter from superintendents), *TN & HR* 19 (August 1897): 157-58; "A Jerseyite and a Graduate" (Letter to the Editor), *TN* 19 (October 1897): 218-19; Lavinia L. Dock, "Trained Nurses Protective Association" (Letter to the Editor), *TN* 18 (May 1897): 279-81; Celia R. Heller, "The N.P.A. Answers" Letter to the Editor, *TN* 18 (June 1897): 337-40; "New York State Legislation," *TN* 24 (January 1900): 55-56. The debate continued in the *American Journal of Nursing:* Josephine Smetsinger, Letter to the Editor, *AJN* 2 (June 1902): 699-700; "A Notice," *AJN* 3 (March 1903): 495. This debate is discussed by Susan Armeny, "Resistance to Professionalization by American Trained Nurses, 1890-1905," paper presented at the Berkshire Conference on the History of Women, 25 August 1978.

27. "Nurses and State Associations," *TN & HR* 46 (January 1911): 30-31; Letter to the Editor, *Pacific Coast Nursing Journal* 10 (March 1914): 130; Ashley, *passim.* Letters in the records of the first nursing registry, the Boston Medical Library Registry of Nurses, also make these points; see Susan Reverby's "Neither for the Drawing Room . . ."

28. Burgess, p. 347; see also Charlotte Aikens, "When is a Probationer Unfit?" *TN & HR* 53 (February 1914): 103-04; "Personal Observation" (Letter to the Editor from a nurse), *TN* 52 (May 1913): 306; M. Adelaide Nutting, "Some Problems of the Training School," *NHR* 12 (November 1908): 6-9.

29. The class background of nursing students is currently being studied by several historians. Nancy Tomes (see note 22) and Jane Mottus, (NYU Dept. of History) from their work on the Philadelphia and New York Hospitals, respectively, suggest that the nursing students, up until World War I, came from middle-class families. My preliminary findings suggest that the smaller schools tended to attract more working-class women and that the shift was, in general, toward working-class women by the 1920s.

30. "Nurses, Patients and Pocketbooks," A paper read at the Annual Convention of Nursing Organizations, Louisville, Kentucky, 7 June 1928, *Bulletin of the American Hospital Association* 2 (July 1928): 300-01.

31. "Overworked Nurses" (Letter to the Editor from a graduate), *TN & HR* 5 (November 1890): 236; "Nurses on Strike," *TN* 26 (February 1901): 95-96; "The Profession Disgraced," *AJN* 3 (April 1903): 592; "Nurses' Strikes," *TN* 19 (September 1902): 235-36; "What is the Remedy," *TN* 37 (July 1906): 36-37; "The Striking Nurse," *TN* 48 (February 1912): 48; "At the Beck of the Walking Delegate," *The Nurse* 1 (October 1914): 308-09; "The Striking Nurse," *TN* 51 (February 1915): 98; "A Trade or a Profession," *TN* 56 (June 1920): 529-30; "Trade Unionism and Nursing," *TN* 56 (March 1920): 240.

32. Hornsby and Schmidt, *passim;* Burgess, *Nurses, Patients and Pocketbooks;* Somerville Hospital School of Nursing, Student Records, Somerville, Mass.; Letters in the Boston Medical Library Registry of Nurses, Rare Book Room, Countway Medical Library.

33. "Labor Turnover in Hospitals," *MH* 21 (August 1923): 159; Charles Neergaard, "Some Causes of Labor Turnover in Hospitals," *MH* 21 (November 1923): 447-48; Edgar Smith, "Why Labor Turnover is Expensive," *MH* (March 1928): 58; Jacob Goodfriend, "How can the Labor Flux Be Brought to an Irreducible Minimum?" *MH* 29 (September 1927): 58; Jacob Goodfriend, "Labor Turnover—What Will the Hospitals Do About It?" *MH* 34 (April 1930): 57, Burgess, pp. 532-33.

34. For a discussion of this in the department stores, see Susan Porter Benson, "The Clerking Sisterhood: Rationalization and the Work Culture of Saleswomen," *Radical America* 12 (March-April 1978): 41-55.

35. L. R. Curtis, "Living Out versus Living In for the Hospital Employees," *MH* 8 (April 1919): 253; "Housing the Personnel," *MH* 26 (March 1924): 205.

36. Morris Hinenberg, "Hospital Property Should not be made PUBLIC," *MH* 60 (March 1943): 88.

37. "Hospital Employees Welfare," *MH* 17 (September 1921): 214; "Welfare Work and Strikes," *MH* 13 (September 1916): 263.

38. S. R. Laycock, "A Basic Need: Personnel Attributes that Satisfy," *Hospitals* 19 (July 1945): 53-54.

39. John Wylley, "Pathways to Better Service Through Proper Training of Employees," *MH* 22 (June 1924): 608.

40. Sallie Jeffries, "The Personnel Problems Must be Put on a Personal Basis," *MH* 60 (May 1943): 55-56; "Discussion—Personnel Problems," *TAHA,* 38th Annual Conference (Cleveland, 1936), p. 821; Burling, pp. 328-333.

41. "Clothes Make the Man," *MH* 20 (April 1923): 376-79; John Bresnahan and Harriet Borman, "A Uniformed Hospital Personnel," *MH* 20 (April 1923): 379.

42. David Montgomery noted that this was particularly common in the rubber and packing industries, but the evidence suggests that the hospitals were not far behind. Discussion with David Montgomery, meeting of the Work Relations Group, Institute for Policy Studies, Washington, D.C., 6 June 1975.

43. "Team Work in the Hospital," *MH* 4 (March 1915): 280; "Another Source of Friction in Hospital Administration," *MH* 6 (February 1916): 112. This phenomenon is discussed in the sociological literature; see, in

223

particular, Robert W. Habenstein and Edwin A. Christ, *Professionalizer, Traditionalizer and Utilizer* (Columbia, Mo., 1955); Everett Hughes et al., *20,000 Nurses Tell Their Story* (Philadelphia, 1958); Virginia Walker, *Nursing and Ritualistic Practice* (New York, 1967).

44. Susan Reverby, "Health: Women's Work," *Prognosis Negative: Crisis in the Health Care System,* edited by David Kotelchuck (New York, 1976), pp. 170-84.

45. Burgess, p. 434.

46. M, "The Attendant, Her Place and Work," *AJN* 20 (November 1919): 154-55; A. K. Haywood, "The Status of the Nursing Attendant," *MH* 19 (September 1922): 226-27; A. C. Jensen, "Training Nursing Attendants," *MH* 51 (November 1938): 68; Winifred Shepler, et al., "Standardized Training Course for Ward Aids," *MH* 51 (December 1938): 68-69; Susan Reverby, "Hospital Organizing in the 1950s: An Interview with Lillian Roberts," *Signs: Journal of Women in Culture and Society* 1 (Summer 1976): 1053-63.

47. I include in this group women whose collective biography has yet to be written: Charlotte Aikens, Mary Riddle, Minnie Goodnow, Anne Goodrich, Shirley Titus, Blanche Pfefferkorn, Eleanor Lambertson.

48. "Why Opinions Differ," *TN & HR* 40 (January 1908): 37-38.

49. It is clear from her remarks that Goodrich was concerned with the standardization of nursing duties, not the hospital standardization movement that was beginning at the same time. "Discussion of the Robert Dickinson paper, 'Hospital Organization as Shown by Charts of Personnel Powers and Functions,' " *Bulletin of the Taylor Society* 3 (October 1917): 8.

50. "Efficiency in the Care of the Patient," *TAHA* 16th Annual Conference (St. Paul, 1914), p. 210.

51. Helen E. Marshall, *Mary Adelaide Nutting, Pioneer of Modern Nursing* (Baltimore, 1972), p. 158. My thanks to Delores Hayden for suggesting that I look at the influences of the home economics movement on nursing.

52. Elizabeth Greener, "A Study of Hospital Nursing Service," *MH* 16 (January 1921): 99-102; A. Owens et. al., "Some Time Studies," *AJN* 27 (February 1927): 99-101; Blanche Pfefferkorn and Marion Rottman, *Clinical Education in Nursing* (New York, 1932); for a review of this literature, see Myrtle Aydelotte, *Nurse Staffing Methodology, A Review and Critique of Selected Literature* (Washington, 1970).

53. Ronda Kotelchuck, "The Depression and the AMA," *Health PAC Bulletin* No. 69 (March/April 1976): 13-18.

54. "National Nursing Groups Appeal to Hospital Trustees," *MH* 34 (July 1932): 108.

55. Malcolm MacEachern, "Which Shall We Choose—Graduate or Student Service," *MH* 38 (June 1932): 94-104; Anna Wolf, "Is the Use of Graduate Nurses for Floor Duty Justified?" *MH* 33 (November 1929): 140-42; "How Many Students can a Graduate Nurse Replace?" *MH* 41 (August 1933): 86; J. C. Geiger, "An Important Change in Policy," *AJN* 32 (February 1932), p. 180.

56. U.S. Bureau of Census, Series B. 192-94.

57. Shirley Titus, "Group Nursing," *AJN* 30 (July 1930): 845-50; Shirley Titus, "Graduate Nursing, The Significance of General Duty Nursing to Our Profession," *AJN* 31 (February 1931): 197-208; Shirley Titus, "Group Nursing and How it Affects the Welfare of the Patient," *MH* 35 (December 1930): 120-28; Subcommittee of the Joint Distribution Committee of the Joint Boards of the Nursing Organizations, "Institutional Nursing," *AJN* 31 (June 1931): 689-92.

58. "What Registries Did," *AJN* 37 (July 1937): 736.

59. Carol Taylor, *In Horizontal Orbit, Hospitals and the Cult of Efficiency* (New York, 1973), p. 58.

60. Burgess, p. 353.

61. Boston Nurses Group, "The False Promise: Professionalism in Nursing," *Science for the People* 10 (May/June 1978): 20-34.

62. Harold E. Smalley and John R. Freeman, *Hospital Industrial Engineering* (New York 1966), p. 49.

63. Pfefferkorn and Rottman, p. 3; Smalley and Freeman, p. 63; Hughes et al.; Aydelotte.

64. Smalley and Freeman, p. 63.

65. Reverby, "Health: Women's Work."

66. David Gaynor, et. al., "RN's Strike: Between the Lines," in Kotelchuck, pp. 229-45.

67. "Roll, Jordan, Roll: A Marx for the Master Class," *Radical History Review* 3 (Summer 1976): 44.

LEON FINK *and*
BRIAN GREENBERG

12 *Organizing Montefiore: Labor Militancy Meets a Progressive Health Care Empire*

I

Among the more dramatic changes in the health services industry during the past twenty years has been the rise of hospital unionism. Employing four times the number of workers in basic steel, hospitals were almost entirely spared the surge of unionization that swept over the nation's major industries during the C.I.O. campaigns of the 1930s and 1940s. Exempted until 1974 from the provisions of the National Labor Relations Act, voluntary, not-for-profit institutions (employing more than two-thirds of all hospital workers) had functioned for years as the low-wage employer of last resort for newly arriving immigrants and southern black and Hispanic migrants to the northern cities. Overwhelmingly female, these moderately skilled service workers toiled in the shadow of the hospitals' physicians and registered nurses (while surpassing them in numbers) as cooks, laundresses, aides, maintenance men, and secretaries. The low status of the hospital work force, its lack of legal bargaining rights, and the philanthropic, humanitarian image of the voluntary institutions (especially the moral sanction against striking helpless patients)

The authors gratefully acknowledge the support of District 1199 National Union of Hospital and Health Care Employees, the Ford Foundation, and the Office of Training and Development of the U. S. Department of Labor for making their research possible. The authors also wish to thank Pamela Brier as well as David Rosner and Susan Reverby for their criticisms of earlier drafts of this essay. An earlier draft of this paper was presented to the Southwest Labor Studies Conference and the Columbia University Seminar in Working Class History.

combined to isolate hospitals from the interest of the country's major labor unions.

In recent years, however, this picture has undergone a marked change. In the decade before 1975, three-quarters of New York City's voluntary hospitals and upwards of 300,000 U.S. hospital workers joined unions.[1] Hospital wages, while still lagging behind the manufacturing sector, passed those of many other service workers during the 1970s. According to the master collective bargaining agreement for New York City voluntary hospitals, the minimum wage alone in January 1978 stood at $190 per week—no princely sum but a far cry from the $28 weekly wage that, as late as 1959, had forced many fully employed hospital workers onto public assistance.

To be sure, unionization alone has not accounted for the increase in earnings and benefits accruing to hospital workers.[2] The workers and their unions have in part benefitted from an astounding boom in the health services industry, an expansion rooted in increasing public expenditures for voluntary hospitals. Since 1950 the proportion of the gross national product spent for health care has nearly doubled, hospital employment has almost tripled, and hospital assets have nearly quadrupled. Among short-term hospitals (voluntary, proprietary [for profit], and state and local governmental), the voluntary, not-for-profit institutions have not only remained the largest but also the fastest growing facilities.[3] One reason is that, instead of paying out dividends to private individuals, the voluntaries plowed back any year-end surplus in the form of new buildings, new technology, and larger physician and administrative salaries. As such, the non-profit sector of the health service industry has demonstrated a capacity for capital consumption, physical expansion, and power and prestige to rival the board rooms of most major corporations.[4] The fuel for these expenditures increasingly has been derived from governmental budgets. While philanthropy and direct payments by patients have fallen drastically since 1950 as sources of health care expenditures, insurance payments (26 percent in 1973) and public subsidy (38 percent in 1973) have accounted for steadily larger shares of the health care pie.[5]

Together, the life-support function of the voluntary hospitals, their centrality to the health care system of large cities, and the role of government itself in the sustenance of these institutions has made almost inevitable the intrusion of the "public"—government officials, press, and organized pressure groups—into the labor-management disputes that have erupted over the past twenty years. The greatest conflicts so far have flared around basic union recognition struggles, capped in 1969 by a 113-day strike by District 1199 in Charleston, South Carolina, in which 1,000 people were arrested. The rise of hospital unions, then, has taken place against a background of expanding hospital wealth and increasing "politicization" of health care institutions. While these factors have no doubt provided new possibilites for organization, they have by no means stilled the traditional resistance by hospital boards of directors to collective bargaining. Today more than eight out of ten voluntary hospital workers remain unorganized and unprotected by union benefits. Nevertheless, the achievement thus far, conditioned by outer developments but generated by the hospital workers themselves, constitutes an important story in contemporary labor and social history. It is a story that has yet to be told.

II

As part of a larger study of hospital workers, we focus here on the first ripple of the recent wave of hospital unionization, namely the organization of Montefiore Hospital in New York City in 1958. While the actors, actions, and decisions at this one hospital were by no means typical (otherwise it might not enjoy its special position within labor history), they do reflect developments that were transforming the industry as a whole. We shall therefore try to set the self-activity of one group of hospital workers in relation to a changing work environment, a developing union organizing strategy, and broader political and cultural influences.

Viewed from afar, Montefiore might long have appeared an attractive prospect for unionization. Under its director, E. M. Bluestone, the hospital, which had been founded as a chronic care home after the Civil War on the site of an infirmary for Confederate prisoners, had gained a reputation in the 1930s and 1940s as a most liberal and innovative institution.[6] Administrators took pride in a "social philosophy" that extended concern for health care "beyond the hospital—into the community."[7] Bluestone brought in Dr. Martin Cherkasky to implement pioneering programs in home care and group practice, and in 1949 he named Cherkasky head of the nation's first hospital-based division of social medicine. As successor to Bluestone in 1950, Cherkasky presided over the final transformation of this center for the "custodial" care of chronic disease into a general hospital.

Part of Montefiore's uniqueness lay in its tolerance of unorthodox political opinion. As a medical resident, Cherkasky himself had been banished from a Philadelphia hospital for trying to organize the house staff. Influenced by the "popular front" ideology of the thirties, Cherkasky continued to think of himself as a radical defender of workers' rights as well as a general menace to the medical establishment. During the McCarthy era Montefiore became somewhat of a haven for left-wing professionals (including several prominent physicians) who could count on protection from outside harassment.

Montefiore's liberalism, however, did not extend to encouragement of union organization among its own work force. At least three times between 1948 and 1958 a core of union sympathizers unsuccessfully attempted campaigns at Montefiore. All three efforts were led by left-wing, white-collar workers in contact with Elliot Godoff, the "father" of New York City hospital unionism.[8] A July 1949 drive by Local 444 of the United Public Workers of America rallied nearly one hundred employees, but the administration ignored the organizers' demands, and the campaign "simply collapsed." While attracting a few blue-collar employees and forcing an end to separate dining rooms for professional, clerical, and service workers, a Teamster (into which the red-baited 444 had been absorbed) effort in 1953 met the same fate. For Montefiore's labor militants in these early years, organizing the hospital formed only one part of a broader commitment to social activism; some of them, for example, joined radical physicians on the staff in trying to rid the surrounding neighborhood of segregated housing.

Why then was it so difficult to organize Montefiore's employees? Our investigation points to fear and division among workers, the general lack of tangible outside support, and a paternalistic management as the main obstacles. In general, liberalism at the top of the hospital structure meant little to the workers at the bottom. None of the workers to whom we spoke—from nurses and lab technicians, to mechanics, cooks, and porters—

cited Montefiore's special social philosophy as reasons why they had taken jobs there or remained at the hospital. Indeed, beneath the enlightened ideals of the directors, personnel policies at Montefiore did not differ much from those at other hospitals. Workers had few rights and were treated in certain respects as dependent members of an extended family. Their "free" meals were deducted in advance from their paychecks, and, as late as the 1950s, some workers continued the old practice of "living in" their place of employment. Employment itself was divided into separate fiefdoms, with departmental supervisors exercising nearly arbitrary authority over their workers. In principle, security was said to be a compensating advantage to the inferior pay of hospital work. But Al Kosloski, who has worked in the engineering (maintenance) department since 1937, remembers that in the pre-union days "your job depended on being cooperative." Unofficially, Kosloski was expected to be available on Saturdays or even on hospital time to help a supervisor or administrator build his driveway or make other home repairs. The supervisors did not hide their anti-union feelings. A hospital messenger who joined the 1953 effort recalls "how hard [it was] for us to get going . . . most of the workers were too scared, afraid to be fired." A Puerto Rican cook put the point more graphically: "White-collar workers are okay . . . [but] if they lost their jobs they could work elsewhere —We belong to our stomachs."

Hierarchical divisions in the hospital were much more complicated than the simple chasm that separated the salaried physicians from the rest of the employees. A set of invidious distinctions of earnings, status, and function also separated nurses, technicians, and the clerical staff from maintenance and service workers. Even within a single department, such as food services, the hierarchy ranged from unskilled dishwashers and pantrymen to skilled craft workers, such as meat-cutters and cooks, to professional dieticians. In earlier years the hospital had encouraged the internalization of hierarchical values with dual facilities for recreation and dining according to employee classification. In part, pride in rank within the hospital became an effective substitute for higher pay, as when licensed practical nurses were required to wear special patches to distinguish them from the higher level registered nurses. In addition, by the 1950s, as older Northern and Eastern European immigrants were replaced by new recruits, the caste of occupation became overlaid by the caste of race—with the lowest paid service sector overwhelmingly black, Puerto Rican, or West Indian. In Montefiore, as in other New York City hospitals, specific ethnic groups, often recruited through familial chain migration patterns, bunched together on a ladder of skill and influence. Even within the housekeeping and food service units, for example, Puerto Ricans predominated in the laundry or in the basement as dishwashers.

Prior to the effort of Local 1199, few Montefiore workers had been convinced of the strength they might derive from unionization. A few politically-minded white-collar workers may have felt part of a movement extending far beyond the hospital, but they had trouble communicating this feeling to the others. A service worker recalled the three earlier attempts at Montefiore only as "some lab workers who used to try to organize us." Al Kosloski remembers the other unions as "not quite strong enough to do anything about the hospitals, [so] we lost faith in them."

Without a union, workers looked for individual solutions to their problems. Dissatisfaction most clearly revealed itself in an astonishing transiency within the hospital labor force, a fact lamented both by hospital administrators and frustrated union organizers alike. In some Montefiore departments turnover rates reached 300 percent per year. Even many veteran hospital workers continued to look on their jobs as temporary expedients. Aside from leaving the hospital altogether (sometimes only to land in another one), the most resourceful of workers had found opportunities for resolving individual grievances and even a degree of upward mobility within the hospital "family." By pitting one supervisor against another or by taking advantage of the liberal solicitude of an administrator, some workers managed to better their lot and create a bit of space for themselves within the hierarchy. Such successes, however, were materially quite limited and required at least an outward acceptance of management's rules of the game.

III

In 1957 Leon Davis launched the Retail Drug Employees, Local 1199, a 6,000-member pharmacists and drugstore employees union rooted in the left-wing industrial unionism of the thirties (and over which Davis had presided almost from its beginnings) on a new mission. In that year Davis recruited Elliot Godoff, recently fired from the Teamsters for his Communist political associations, for yet another assault on New York City's hospitals. After a frustrating start among several proprietary institutions, Godoff turned to the voluntaries and chose Montefiore, where he had a few long-standing contacts and which had a unique administration, as his first target. Over the course of a prolonged campaign from December 1957 to August 1958, the organizers signed up a majority of Montefiore's 900 workers (excluding the registered nurses). The next phase of the campaign embraced an elaborate set of maneuvers—involving the city government and the Central Labor Council, as well as a strike threat—to force recognition from the administrators, which finally came on 7 December 1958. The workers ratified the agreement, selecting Local 1199 as their bargaining agent. In March 1959 the union negotiated its first Montefiore contract, an achievement that quickly reverberated throughout the city. Six months later 3,500 workers walked out in an unprecedented 46-day strike at seven of the city's major voluntary hospitals. This confrontation ended in a standoff agreement stopping short of formal recognition but providing grievance and arbitration machinery that allowed the union a crucial "foot in the door." As a result of coordinated work place and political pressure, New York City hospital workers finally gained collective bargaining rights when they were enrolled under the state labor relations act in 1963. This achievement, a direct legacy of the Montefiore events five years before, led directly to the organization of the mass of New York City hospital workers.

In looking first at the internal mobilization of the Montefiore work force, the relevant question is: Why did 1199's effort of 1958 succeed where three others had failed? Our work points to the following levels of explanation: (1) changes in work relations within the hospital, (2) cultivation of feelings of group pride and strength among the service workers, and (3) integration of the union's presence with indigenous work group leaders.

A managerial revolution accompanied Montefiore's transformation into a general hospital. To instill greater efficiency and productivity in its operations, Montefiore (in a pattern common to other hospitals) installed men with outside business experience to direct the expansion and modernization of support services.[9] Two such experts of the early 1950s unintentionally helped to stimulate the union drive. Irving Stern proudly introduced a "profit-and-loss" consciousness into the laundry operations. Early in 1958 he installed a 500-pound washer and a flatwork ironer that handled 1,900 sheets and towels per hour. Jacques Bloch joined Dr. Cherkasky's food service department in 1954 with a background in hotel and business administration. Within three years Bloch had centralized the dishwashing and tray-assembly systems, opened a new cafeteria, and, with the attitude that "food is money," eliminated the paternalistic "free food" system, thus increasing the amount of take-home money in workers' pay envelopes. Yet it was precisely against these two "modernizers" that the resentments of unionizing workers centered. Workers dubbed Stern "the Bull" for his dictatorial manner and complained that Bloch was personally "remote" and that his task supervision interfered with a pre-established, more casual "workers' way of life."

In short, the "progressive" refurbishing of Montefiore's personnel policies, which by the administrators' yardstick offered tangible gains to hospital workers, appeared to many workers as nothing more than closer supervision and harassment on the job. As a result of such grievances, union appeals to work place "dignity" and "respect" fell on all the more attentive ears. It was no coincidence, therefore, that the kitchen and laundry staffs became bulwarks of the 1199 drive.

Local 1199's organizing campaign did not ignore existing divisions and stratifications among hospital workers; instead, it turned this apparent obstacle to the union's advantage. The process of organization worked by seeking a kind of coalition of distinct social groups within the hospital. Although Godoff called on some of his old left-wing friends at Montefiore in charting the 1199 drive, the effort was concentrated from the beginning among the service and blue-collar workers. A hospital mortician active in an earlier drive observed that "the 1958 effort was left to the newcomers." Leaflets appealed to workers by departments—"special Meeting of the Nutrition Dept.," "Attention PN's and Nurses Aides," etc. The union also adapted to the racial realities at Montefiore, assigning Theodore Mitchell, a former drugstore porter and the drug union's first black officer to full-time duty at Montefiore alongside Godoff. Similarly, these two chief organizers tapped Salvatore Cordero, a messenger in the nursing unit, to "try to get in touch with your boys (i.e., the Spanish-speaking workers)." When twenty Puerto Rican workers braved a thunderstorm to attend an early organizing meeting, the union leaders knew for the first time that they stood a real chance. In part, Local 1199 benefited from the same gathering cohesiveness across skill and occupational lines within the minority communities that would soon energize the civil rights movement. The Montefiore workers' cause was taken up by black politicians and ministers and by Harlem's *Amsterdam News*. In the Spanish-speaking community, *El Diario* also supported "La Cruzada de Local 1199."

Finally, the organizing campaign worked because the union was able to inspire workers with a tangible sense of what they might win and to harness individual ambitions to a project for collective advancement. The assignment of drugstore stewards to the Montefiore picket lines, the opening of an office across from the hospital, and the scheduling of key meetings at the union's Manhattan headquarters were all calculated to transfer a sense of the union's collective strength to the unorganized workers. Initial courtship by the union staff gathered to their cause some exceptionally motivated individuals who in turn carried the union message to their fellow workers. Thelma Bowles, a black licensed practical nurse who would become a general organizer for 1199 after her performance in the Montefiore campaign, was drawn to the union by her disgust over the hospital's insistence on insignia patches. She may also have been motivated by a drive for self-improvement stirred by parents who had always urged her to go into business or to become a school teacher.

As a group, the active core of organizers was drawn less from alienated rebels than from workers who enjoyed their work, received good marks from their supervisors, and had shown a talent for job advancement within their skill categories. For Al Kosloski, who came from a Polish family of hard-coal miners near Wilkes-Barre, Pennsylvania, participation in unions was a natural part of working-class life. But Kosloski had also exploited his individual opportunities to their limit, transferring from an initial job as pantryman to a job as gardener and assistant head gardener. Kosloski then parlayed World War II service into the training he needed to begin his pursuit of an engineering license, and today his supervisor regards him as "one of the best engineers in the plant." "My dream," said Kosloski, "was to move up, keep movin' up." This was the man who organized the "Four Horsemen" in the maintenance department to spread the union word. Kenneth Downes, a native of Barbados with an island background as fisherman, butler, carpenter, barman, painter and merchant seaman before he took a job as dishwasher at Montefiore in 1950, also worked his way up by the rules. To pick up extra money he would run the bar at doctors' dances, and his West Indian cooking soon won him a raise in position and salary from his supervisors. Working the morning grill, Downes took pride in getting the staff off to a good day; with uncommon care, he cleaned the grill with his "spade" after each egg, then applied fresh lard. A series of confrontations between Downes and Bloch, the new food service director, began when Bloch reduced the operating hours of the grill. To avoid his dismissal, a friendly woman in personnel transferred Downes in 1957 to the safety and traffic department. Circulating through the hospital on guard duty, Downes signed up more workers for the union in 1958 than any other individual. Following his retirement, Downes returned to Barbados to live, but on a recent visit to New York he recalled his fatherlike role in the unionization campaign: "All I wanted is for my poor workers to get a proper salary. . . . I fought, I walked all night with cards in my pocket getting them signed up and the bottom of my shoes burnin' like hot peppers." As individuals, Bowles, Kosloski, and Downes commanded the respect of the hospital workers; by their actions, they made it possible for other individuals to think of getting ahead by getting behind the union.

Relying on these and other work place militants, Local 1199 generated an effective organizing drive at Montefiore. By August 1958, some 500 of Montefiore's 900 workers had signed union cards. Although very weak in the nursing division (except for the aides and orderlies) and in the laboratory and clerical departments, 1199 signed up overwhelming majorities in the housekeeping, food service, traffic and safety, and engineering departments. In most work places a union with such backing might have begun to rejoice, but any celebration of a union victory here was premature. The union majority was without legal force; under existing labor law, the hospital could, and would, ignore the organization of its workforce. Of necessity, therefore, the union next undertook to do battle for recognition and a contract—an engagement with its own logic, played out over a quite different terrain from that of the organizing drive.

IV

Formal recognition of 1199 as the bargaining agent for the Montefiore workers, it appears in retrospect, depended on: (1) continued work place militancy, (2) pressure from the public (in particular, the press, the liberal community, and organized labor), (3) managerial ambivalence at Montefiore, the result of a conflict between the hospital's liberal self-conception and its resistance to trade unionism, and (4) compensating financial inducements. Although militancy and the public appeal were vital to keeping the union recognition campaign alive, they were not sufficient in themselves to overcome hospital resistance. It is the latter two elements that appear to have been most critical to the ultimate settlement. Yet it is harder to specify just how these operated. What we shall do here is to set down the details of each component and suggest the possible ways they collectively brought about a negotiated settlement recognizing the union's presence at Montefiore.

To maintain and make use of their internal hospital majority, the union troops had, above all, to remain active. Davis recognized that signed union cards were not enough, Local 1199 had to "test the worker's discipline." A conspicuous, although most often symbolic, protest at the hospital persisted for months. As Godoff told the 1199 Executive Council on 22 September 1958, during the summer the workers had become "very restless . . . [They] appear ready for action and look to us for leadership." Betty Rosoff, a lab technician who had been active in the earlier union drives, points out, "The feeling was [that] this was our chance and we should make the most of it."

Following the election of stewards and the development of a union infrastructure at Montefiore by the end of summer 1958, Local 1199 carefully began to test the depth of its support. Workers were called on to march with signs and pass out leaflets during their off hours (before and after work or during lunch), although they were not asked to actually walk off their jobs.

236

Widespread participation in these activities not only indicated the union's strength but also helped to provide, as Davis notes, "*personal contact* with [the] union." Moe Foner, 1199's executive secretary, recalling his idea to have a petition in the form of a big poster positioned in front of the hospital, observed: "[It] gives people confidence once their names are down in public . . . [and] strengthens resolve." Such demonstrations of solidarity continued throughout the "long wait of summer." But the hospital's management was still "sitting tight" and was taking "no action regarding the workers."

Recognizing, as Moe Foner says, that we "couldn't beat the hospital ourselves," Local 1199 worked to stimulate outside pressure. In a campaign conducted "like a crusade . . . good versus evil," Foner enlisted the support of James Wechsler of the *New York Post,* together with the editors of the *Amsterdam News* and *El Diario,* and in Davis' name, appealed to the informal authority of the *New York Times.* Hospital administrators soon found the depressing economic condition of the hospital workers spread out before them in the daily press. This appeal to public moral sympathy and sense of fair play extended to letters sent to Eleanor Roosevelt, Senator Herbert H. Lehman, and others "on behalf of 600 Negro and Puerto Rican workers . . . [who are] terribly exploited and are practically desperate unless something is done in their behalf." The recipients were asked to use their "great influence to persuade Mr. Victor Riesenfeld, President of the Board of Directors of Montefiore Hospital, to sit down with a committee of the union and attempt to work out some of the problems."

Such personal entreaties were effective. In her syndicated column, "My Day," Eleanor Roosevelt commented on the severe hardship faced by hospital workers, and both she and Lehman wrote personally to Riesenfeld. Perhaps Moe Foner is right when he states that though in her actions Roosevelt was very cautious, "the very fact that she said something made what we were doing important." Yet the letters to Riesenfeld seem to have been written more as gentle advice, reflecting the prevailing friendship network among a socially prominent elite, than as strong protests in support of union recognition. In this spirit, in a handwritten aside to his letter to Riesenfeld, Lehman added his wife's personal regards and expressed the hope that "in spite of your many duties you still find time for your family."

A key factor in broadening the base of Local 1199's efforts at Montefiore was the support it received from organized labor and, in particular, Harry Van Arsdale, president of New York City's Central Labor Council. Van Arsdale had to overcome the reluctance of some trade unionists to accept the legitimacy of organizing hospitals as well as the unionists' fears of 1199's maverick past. For Van Arsdale, however, the hospital campaign offered a dramatic test of organized labor's power and good intentions with regard to the city's newest working-class population (and it also avoided the thorny complications of black entry into established "white" organized trades). Beginning with the Montefiore effort, Van Arsdale employed the considerable political resources at his command to pressure city officials (including his friend, Mayor Robert F. Wagner) towards a peaceful resolution of the Montefiore dispute. Davis feels that "Harry looks at us, rightly so . . . as [a] good part of his own achievement."

Continued worker militancy and the growing public campaign kept the union drive alive but brought no immediate resolution to the struggle. Administrative intransigency stemmed at least in part from an awareness that the confrontation with Local 1199 involved more than local stakes. Recognition of the union at Montefiore would be the first major breakthrough in the history of hospital organizing. Victor Weingarten, coordinator of Montefiore's public relations, remembers being warned by other hospital directors of a continuous escalation of demands and the loss of administrative control should the union be recognized at the institution. Indeed, the idea of unionization struck even the liberal Cherkasky as an imposition on legitimate managerial prerogatives. Anti-union letters from donors to the Federation of Jewish Philanthropies, with which Montefiore was vitally associated, also convinced Weingarten that "it would be difficult to get philanthropic money if [we then appear to] give it all to unions."

The opposition of Montefiore's own board of trustees, however, was an even more critical obstacle to union recognition. Composed of bank directors, corporate attorneys, and industrial executives (including the publisher of the liberal *Nation* magazine)—men accustomed to dealing with unions as an inevitable but unenjoyable part of the private "business" world—the board naturally found the special non-union sanctum of the hospitals (to use Cherkasky's word) "heavenly."

Nevertheless, there was a tension between these anti-union sentiments and traditional notions of Jewish philanthropy, especially given the social idealism avowed by Cherkasky and his staff. In fact, Cherkasky alleges, it is this factor that overcame his resistance to the union and led to its recognition. He recalls that, as the weeks dragged by without any change in the hospital's position, Davis wrote appealing to him as a man of "good will." In this letter of 28 November 1958, Davis admitted to Cherkasky that a policy of complete recalcitrance on management's part "could destroy the union." He wondered, however, whether Montefiore's director would "rightly participate in this concerted effort to defeat these workers [and] destroy their hopes for better conditions now and in the future. . . . The question still remains whether that [a union defeat] solves any problems for the management, for the workers, or for you who must assume a great share of the burden." Flattering Cherkasky as "the most important factor in this whole situation," Davis implored him to take the steps necessary to avoid an ugly strike, to side with "reason against insanity." Looking back on these events, Cherkasky calls the Davis letter the "final blow—there wasn't a chord in me that Leon didn't strike." In the director's opinion, the letter "turned the whole thing around," Cherkasky resolved to end the stalemate, and he soon persuaded Victor Riesenfeld, president of the board of trustees, that "if we win, we lose—we do not want to be a part of that."

It is difficult to assess just what the impact of Cherkasky's "crisis of conscience" may have been. His reminiscences might be dismissed as romantic, especially given the outcome, an attempt to put himself on the side of the angels. Yet it is clear from Davis's letter, as well as from the whole tone of the campaign to create public pressure on Montefiore, that the union consciously shaped its appeals to provoke such a crisis. And for Cherkasky, at least, to deny the union was to deny the image he held of himself as a sensitive and visionary administrator.

Clearly, even before Cherkasky had decided to deal openly with Local 1199, he had recognized limits beyond which he was unwilling to go in resisting the union. Union organizers, for example, were astounded at the ease with which they could penetrate the hospital, sometimes communicating with workers even when supervisors were in the same room. Sarah Goldstein, Montefiore's director of volunteer services, recalls the day when Pinkerton guards arrived to protect the hospital from union picketers demonstrating at noon time. The employment (apparently by an administrative subordinate) of this notorious union-busting firm—one to which Jewish liberals of the thirties would have had an instinctual revulsion—"shocked" Mrs. Goldstein: when she sought out the director, she found Cherkasky so embarrassed by the episode that he ordered the guards removed, "and they were gone in twenty minutes."

On balance, then, we can recognize the importance (and historical legitimacy) of the ideological factor in bringing Montefiore to heel. Yet financial calculations also figured prominently, if somewhat elusively, in Montefiore's ultimate accommodation with the union. From the moment of his original discussions with Riesenfeld concerning union recognition, Cherkasky linked a settlement with an increase in the reimbursement rate paid by the city to the voluntary hospitals for ward patients.[10] In making this connection, the director displayed a long-range astuteness regarding the hospital's future growth. Clearly, as he and other "progressives" realized, neither private philanthropy, like that from the Federation of Jewish Philanthropies, nor fees for service could alone provide the capital necessary for the extensive changes that the hospital was undergoing and projected for the future. Rather, some means had to be found to increase public funding to voluntary hospitals and make government a bigger participant in health care.

In fact, Cherkasky claimed, in a 1959 *Modern Hospital* article, besides the hospital's concern for managerial prerogatives, Montefiore's resistence to unionization was premised on a belief that "Organization was meaningless without some method by which the hospital could provide funds to cover potential wage increases." In the years to come, the Montefiore director proved exceptionally able at devising several such effective methods. From the mid-1950s through the next decade, Montefiore, according to one study, financed a fourfold increase in plant size. As early as 1961, Cherkasky helped to establish an affiliation agreement between the voluntary hospitals and private medical colleges to staff the municipal hospitals of the City of New York. For its services to publicly owned Morrisania Hospital (since closed), Montefiore received $7 million. During the decade the Montefiore Hospital complex became the largest employer in the Bronx as its energetic director attracted major federal grants both for research and community medicine.[11] In retrospect, therefore, Cherkasky's bargain with the city at the height of the union fight, seems to have unlocked the financial secret to successful hospital management for the ensuing period.

At least in this one way, therefore, unionization appears to have played a role in the construction of modern, rationalized, voluntary hospital-medical school complexes (or "health care empires" as they have been called), which have come not only to dominate health care delivery in American cities but to assume an increasing proportion of tax dollars. To conclude that Cherkasky turned the "threat" of unionization into an agent of hospital expansionism, however, is not to attribute to him Machiavellian genius from the outset of Montefiore's labor troubles. The settlement there was indeed a breakthrough in voluntary hospital financing, but its implications could not have been fully predicted in the years before Medicare and Medicaid. Rather, it is more plausible to assume that once he had (privately) made the "big" decision of 1958, that is, to abide by a union election at Montefiore, Cherkasky did his best to sweeten the decision.

The subsidy, it seems clear, was not the major sticking point in reaching an accord with the union at Montefiore. As Mayor Wagner (who appeared then to have miraculously resolved the conflict by coming up with money for the hospital in the nick of time) himself recalls the situation, the money issue was not central: "You can always find a little more here or there—that's not a very big problem once you've got it [the basic agreement] going." The crux of the matter was ideological and political: whether Montefiore would become the first major hospital to sacrifice part of its managerial prerogatives and yield to union pressure. Indeed, so controversial was the principle of union recognition that, even after making up his own mind, President of the Board Riesenfeld (according to Weingarten) waited to bring the conflict to a crisis point in order to show Montefiore's financial patrons as well as other anxious hospitals that Montefiore had not simply "caved in" to union demands.

In the first week of December 1958 the situation reached just such a point. On December 3 the union met and set the following Monday, December 8, at 6 a.m. as the strike deadline. Faced with the unwelcome prospect of confrontation, Mayor Wagner, at the urging of both Riesenfeld and Van Arsdale, called an emergency meeting to negotiate a settlement. With Van Arsdale representing the union's interests, they reached agreement only hours before the deadline. The hospital would recognize Local 1199 as "the sole collective bargaining agent pending a certification election and negotiate an agreement dealing with all issues."

Publicly the issue of the subsidy remained unsettled, but privately the city agreed to raise, as of 1 July 1959, its support of ward patients in the voluntary hospitals from $16 per day to $20 per day. On 30 December 1958 a union election was held at Montefiore. Of some 900 workers eligible to vote, 608 chose Local 1199 as their bargaining agent; only 30 opposed it. Early in 1959 the union and the hospital began negotiations, and by March they had initialed a contract. In themselves, the terms represented modest gains: a $30 monthly increase in pay, time-and-one-half pay for work above a 40-hour week, establishment of grievance procedures, and the setting of minimum provisions for sick leave and vacation time. More importantly perhaps, the contract offered visible proof of the power of organization: A union among hospital workers had begun.

For all its extraordinary principals and despite its sublimated climax, the organization of Montefiore Hospital foreshadowed some important themes for contemporary health institutions and their labor forces. We have documented here how a "new" working-class population, outside the traditional reach of trade unionism, effectively mobilized as management rationalized a growing health empire. We have stressed the immediate public and political nature of hospital organizing and likewise its dependence on a favorable outside political balance of power, as well as on a militant display of strength by workers in hospital labs, kitchens, laundries, and boiler rooms. Finally, we have highlighted the impact of managerial ideology and financial factors on the outcome of hospital-labor conflict and, in so doing, have related unionism itself to the basic dilemmas facing health policy makers in the present day.

Notes

1. The most active unions in the hospital field today include the Service Employees International Union, especially strong on the West Coast, which claimed 140,000 members in 1974; District 1199, National Union of Hospital and Health Care Employees, with nearly 80,000 members in 1974, three-quarters of whom were located in New York City, New Jersey, and Connecticut; and the American Federation of State, County, and Municipal Employees (AFSCME), whose impact has been widespread in publicly owned hospitals across the country (Jonathan Rivin, "The Impacts of Unionization on Unskilled Hospital Workers and the Hospital Industry" [Senior honors thesis, Harvard College, 1977], p. 50).

2. Recent studies by labor economists place the positive union versus non-union wage and fringe differential for hospital workers at a modest 6-8 percent. Such studies undoubtedly have a conservative bias, however, in that at most they can compare pay scales at a given moment or several moments. They are inherently unable (because the process is not quantifiable) to assess the importance of unionization as one factor in a complex historical evolution of the wage. See Roger Feldman and Richard M. Scheffler, "The Effect of Labor Unions on Hospital Employees Wages," paper presented to the Southern Economic Association, New Orleans, 3 November 1977; also Myron D. Fottler, "The Union Impact on Hospital Wages," *Industrial and Labor Relations Review*, Spring 1977, pp. 345-59.

3. Leonard Rodberg and Gelvin Stevenson, "The Health Care Industry in Advanced Capitalism," *Review of Radical Political Economy* 9 (Spring 1977): 110; American Hospital Association, *Hospital Statistics, 1971.* Hospital expansion was computed on the basis of the increase in the number of beds; since 1950 the voluntaries have grown by 86 percent by this measure, state and municipals by 46 percent, and proprietaries by 26 percent.

4. Rodberg and Stevenson, p. 109.

5. Rivin, Tables 1-3, p. 9. National benchmarks in the trend toward public underwriting of the private non-profit hospitals were the Hill-Burton Hospital Survey and Construction Act of 1946 and the Medicare and Medicaid programs enacted in 1966.

6. Health-PAC, "Empire Survey (II) Einstein-Montefiore: Bronxmanship," *Health-PAC Bulletin*, April 1969.

7. Further direct quotations in text derive either from oral interviews conducted by the authors in 1975-1977 or from District 1199 archives located at the Labor-Management Documentation Center, New York School of Industrial and Labor Relations, Cornell University.

8. While working as a pharmacist at Maimonides Hospital in the late forties and enjoying good relations with its administration, Godoff secured a union contract, the first of its kind for New York City hospital workers.

9. Looking back over Montefiore's evolution from a chronic care to a general hospital, Cherkasky described the change as a difference between "slow motion and speed up." In the old days hospital admissions could be measured in terms of a couple hundred patients a year; "now we admit 150 patients a day." The "personnel, facility, active pace—the whole institution [underwent a] cataclysmic change." For a more detailed discussion

of changing hospital management practices, see Susan Reverby's unpublished paper, written in 1975, "Borrowing a Volume from Industry, Hospital Management Reform 1900-1945."

10. Montefiore sought a city guarantee to raise the $16 per day reimbursement rate paid voluntary hospitals for ward patients to the $27 per day rate paid to municipal hospitals. The indigent patients had become an increasing factor in the hospital's operations, as more and more of the Bronx was transformed into the nation's most miserable ghetto.

11. Health-PAC, "Empire Survey (II) Einstein-Montefiore Bronxmanship."

PART V

PERSONAL HEALTH
AND PUBLIC POLICY

In the 1970s we have witnessed a resurgence in the insistence on personal responsibility for health care. This concern is the health sector's analogue of the "rugged individualism" ethic. Clearly the ethic has two sides: self-help and victim-blaming. In this article Robert Crawford addresses both of these ideologies and analyzes the forces that have led to their recent reemergence.

As other articles in this volume have argued, during periods of uncertainty health often becomes a critical metaphor for other concerns. In the nineteenth century, Verbrugge has shown, middle-class women organized an institute to learn about self-care; now, Crawford argues, this impulse is being transformed from ideology to policy within a new political and social context.

This chapter on contemporary policy raises historical questions. What are the economic and political reasons behind the emergence of a concern with personal health or dependence on professionals at different historical moments? How does the concern with personal health become victim-blaming? Does this form of analysis shed light on earlier examples of medical controversy on the "over-use" or "abuse" of medical care?

ROBERT CRAWFORD

13 *Individual Responsibility and Health Politics in the 1970s*

Medical services and health have always been objects of intense ideological activity. As valued resources, as indicators of individual and social well-being or malaise, as mirrors of fundamental social divisions, they have the quality of projecting and spotlighting the deepest conflicts of American life. Like other critical sectors, medicine and health are symbolic of a continuing crisis of the social order. That such a crisis exists—and that it is at once economic, political, and ideological—is a basic premise on which the following argument is based.

Most simply stated, the crisis of medicine and health in the late 1970s takes two forms: (1) the tension between a medical system that has become incredibly costly and an expanded popular expectation of rights to medical services and (2) the tension between ineffective medical services and a growing awareness of the social causation of disease.

Both aspects of the current crisis have jumped the boundaries of the medical sector itself. Dominant economic and political interests are threatened by the failure to find a solution in the routine processes of health politics. Activity aimed at resolving the tensions on a symbolic level will be the focus here. The analysis suggests that the ideological response would direct attention away from the threatening aspects of the crisis and at

For helpful comments and editorial suggestions, mostly on an earlier draft, thanks to Evan Stark, Susan Reverby, John McKnight, Nancy Hartsock, Sol Levine, Cathy Stepanek, Isaac Balbus, and participants in the East Coast Health Discussion Group. I am especially indebted to Lauren Crawford who provided many hours in discussion and in preparation of this manuscript.

the same time facilitate solutions that are compatible with the political and economic agendas of dominant interests, particularly large corporate capital.

The Challenge to Medicine

During the last twenty years, and especially in the last decade, we have witnessed a remarkable expansion in the health sector. The expansion has been powered by a growth coalition able to win the extension of employee health benefits, the socialization of costs for the aged and many of the poor, and the direct subsidization of medical research, provider, and training institutions. Sustained development of the economy fed and enabled that growth. Government expenditures, private insurance premiums, and corporate investments provided the capital. In the course of its growth, medicine has come to capture the imagination, hope, and pocketbooks of the American public. The medical enterprise as a whole has enjoyed an almost complete absence of opposition. There has been a consistent demand for more.

In recent years, however, the hegemony of medicine has been challenged. First, reflective of political tensions pervading the entire society in the 1960s, medical institutions and practices were faced with opposition to destructive institutional expansion in ghetto areas, protests against a tiered delivery system that relegates the poor and minorities to inferior and less accessible services, and conflicts over control of the "Great Society" health programs. But none of these conflicts questioned the essential value of medicine. The problems were most often identified as access and equity, and the solutions were seen in terms of new, neighborhood-targeted services, expanded governmental benefits, institutional reform, and citizen participation and control. In the more quiescent 1970s the legacy of these struggles is manifest in occasional organized resistence to cutbacks of benefits, conflict over control of health systems agencies, an increased popular support for national health insurance or service.

In the late 1960s and early 1970s a second challenge emerged from the women's movement, which criticized professional male authority over women's lives and simultaneously raised the issue of overmedicalization. Feminists argued that medicine was sexist in diagnosis, in treatment, and in its very conception of female pathology. Seen as an institution of social control, medicine was assailed for perpetuating dependency and negative self-images among women.[1] Women's self-help groups and alternative women's clinics were organized. Segments of the broader self-help movement picked up many of these themes, developed a critique of overmedicalization and espoused a goal of individual autonomy.

A third trend has, for the first time, brought to the forefront of public discussion the issues of overmedicalization, medical effectiveness, and the importance of non-therapeutic determinants of health. Unlike the previous challenges, this is not primarily a grassroots phenomenon. Although an amalgam of a wide variety of groups—including self-helpers, non-medical healers/entrepreneurs, and those with specific disease interests—have raised these issues, this development emanated from the academic world, foundations, and, to some extent, government agencies.

First, impressive evidence on the relative ineffectiveness of medicine in reducing mortality and morbidity has been added to the academic literature and has been popularized in this country by Illich, Fuchs, and Carlson.[2] A profusion of conferences, articles, and media coverage has shifted debate within the health policy field from a concern with issues of access and equality to questions of the relevance or the limits of medicine for maintaining health. The Rockefeller Foundation, Blue Cross Association, and the Health Policy Program of the University of California, for example, sponsored a conference linking critiques of medical effectiveness with an examination of alternative strategies for maintaining health, especially change in individual behavior and the practice of a myriad of activities grouped under the concept of "holistic medicine."[3] Similar themes are now emerging with regularity in symposiums on cost control, in meetings of professional associations, and in the press. Finally, concrete policy recommendations for a reorientation from medical care to health promotion have generated considerable interest and, as will be seen below, have already been translated into public policy. Everywhere the assertion can be heard that the medical system is a bloated giant that needs to be contained and even subdued. In short, medicine confronts a number of critiques ranging from what has been called "therapeautic nihilism" to more modest proposals for therapeutic constraint.[4] Together they may constitute the most serious challenge to medicine since the pre-Flexnerian period.

But much more is at stake than the unquestioned enchantment with medicine, for the contention also is being made that, although health is a complex matter and therefore requires several kinds of efforts, individual responsibility is the key ingredient. In place of admittedly expensive and ineffective medical services, it is said, individual change must be the focus of the nation's efforts to promote and maintain health. People should use the medical system less and instead adopt healthy lifestyles; or, as it was declared by one pundit, "living a long life is essentially a do-it-yourself proposition." These assertions perform the function of *blaming the victim.* They avert any serious discussion of social or environmental factors and instead locate the problem of poor health and its solution in the individual. Further, they imply, sometimes explicitly, that since people's own misbehavior is the heart of the problem of health and illness, people should *demand less* medical care. Rights and entitlements for access to medical services are almost by definition now considered inappropriate. Thus, in becoming a premise for public policy, these pronouncements are providing the material for a new public philosophy by which problems are defined and answers proposed.

Similar ideologies of individual responsibility have always been popular among providers and academics trying to justify inequality in the utilization of medical services. During the period of rapid expansion in the health sector, higher morbidity and mortality rates for the poor and minorities were explained by emphasizing their lifestyle habits, especially their health and utilization behavior. These "culture of poverty" explanations emphasized delay in seeking medical help, resistance to medical authority, and reliance on unprofessional folk healers or advisors. As Catherine Riessman summarizes:

> According to these researchers, the poor have undergone multiple negative experiences with organizational systems, leading to avoidance behavior, lack of trust, and hence a disinclination to seek care and follow medical regimens except in dire need.[5]

Now, in a period of fiscal crisis and cost control, the same higher morbidity rates and demands for more access through comprehensive national health insurance are met with a barrage of statements about the limits of medicine and the lack of appropriate health behavior. Several commentators now link overuse by the poor with their faulty health habits. Again, education is seen as the solution. Previously the poor were blamed for not using medical services enough, for relying too much on their own resources, for undue suspicion of modern medicine. Now they are blamed for relying too much on medical services and not enough on their own resources. In both cases, of course, structural factors are rarely mentioned; but structural factors are behind this ideological shift.

The Crisis of Costs

The cost crisis is transforming the entire political landscape in the health sector. What makes inflation in the health sector so critical in the 1970s is not only its spectacular rate but also its concurrence with wider economic and fiscal crises. We now face a situation in which inflation and expenditures for human services have become the primary targets of a strategy aimed at restoring "optimal conditions" for investment and growth in the corporate sector. The costs of medical services to government have aggravated a fiscal crisis in which the direction of public spending is the issue and raising taxes is considered inimical to corporate priorities. Further, high medical costs have become a direct threat to the corporate sector in two important ways: first, by adding significantly to the costs of production through increases in health benefit settlements with labor; and, second, by diverting consumer expenditures from other corporate products. The fact that large corporations have extensively invested in medical and health-related products does not significantly alter this picture.

The costs of production for corporations are being dramatically affected by increases in benefit settlements. General Motors claims it spent more money with Blue Cross and Blue Shield in 1975 than it did with U.S. Steel, its principal supplier of metal. Standard Oil of Indiana announced that employee health costs for the corporation had tripled over the past seven years.[6] Chrysler estimates that in 1976 it paid $1,500 per employee for medical benefits or a total of $205 million in the United States. "Unlike most other labor costs that can and do vary with the

251

level of production," the corporation complains, "medical costs continue to rise in good times as well as bad."[7] The implications for consumer costs are obvious. General Motors added $175 to the price of every car and truck by passing on its employee medical benefit costs. In a period in which consumption and investment are stalled, while foreign competition adds an additional barrier to raising prices, such figures are startling. Corporate and union leaders are expressing in every possible forum their concern over the impact of rising medical costs upon prices, wages, and profits.

Thus, substantial political pressures are being mobilized to cut the direct costs to corporations and to cut the indirect costs of social programs generally. The politics of growth that dominated the previous period are giving way to the politics of curbing that growth in the present period. Just a few years ago the political emphasis was on increasing utilization. Now it is on reducing utilization. Besides regulatory measures, the strategies being adopted include cutbacks in public programs, especially Medicaid, and public hospitals and a shifting of the burden of costs back to employees, old people, and consumers in general.[8] In addition, corporations, often with the participation of unions, are adopting new internal strategies aimed at curbing costs.[9]

Most important is the growing consensus among corporate and governmental leaders that comprehensive national health insurance is unacceptable at current cost levels. In his campaign for the presidency, Jimmy Carter, aware of its popular appeal and importance to organized labor, committed himself to a comprehensive insurance program; but, in reminding the nation in April 1977 that balancing the budget by 1981 is his paramount domestic goal, Carter warned that the costs of such a program would be prohibitive. Secretary of Health, Education, and Welfare, Joseph Califano, more explicitly argued that cost control is a necessary precondition for national health insurance or "some other system."[10] These and numerous other signs indicating that the prospects for comprehensive insurance are receding behind a shield of rhetoric and a language of gradualism.

Popular Demand for the Extension of Rights and Entitlements

In order to understand the importance of a new ideology that tells people they must rely less on the medical system and more on themselves, the cost crisis must be viewed in the context of the legacy of the preceding period, a time in which popular expectations of medicine and political demands for unhindered access to medical services reached their highest levels. Growth reinforced those expectations, as did years of propaganda by a medical and research establishment strengthened by occasional but spectacular medical successes. Medicine was promoted in almost religious terms, a promise of deliverance from pain and illness and even a "death of death."

For years people were conditioned to believe in the value of consuming high levels of medical services and products. At a time when these beliefs became celebrated cultural values, large numbers of people continued to experience difficulty in obtaining regular access to primary care services and faced financial disaster for unusual medical expenses. Access came to be considered an essential component of family and personal security and an integral part of the wage bargain for organized labor. The idea of medical care as a right became widely accepted in a period in which rights were forced onto the political agenda of the nation. By the early 1970s popular pressures for national health insurance began to swell. As benefits shrink in the face of uncontrollable inflation, the sentiment for a comprehensive program continues to build.

Now, however, just at the point when medical care has become broadly viewed as a right and there is a growing demand for the extension of entitlements, people are suddenly being pressured to use the system less. If people are to modify their expectations, if their demands for guaranteed access are to be sidetracked, and if legislators and other policymakers are to be convinced of the necessity for retrenchment, a new ideology must be developed to replace the unquestioned power of medicine and to break the link between the provision of services and popular political demands. People will not relinquish their expectations unless their belief in medicine as a panacea is broken and the value of access is replaced with a new preoccupation with boot-strapping activities aimed at controlling at-risk behaviors. In a political climate of fiscal, energy, and cost crises, self-sacrifice and self-discipline emerge as popular themes. In lieu of rights and entitlements, individual responsibility, self-help and holistic health move to the center of discussion.[11]

253

The Politics of Retrenchment

The flavor of the ideology is evident in the comments of some of its more explicit proponents. Both direct policy proposals and indirect policy implications are abundant. With an implied attack on social programs, for example, Victor Fuchs, a noted health economist, writes: "Some future historian, in reviewing mid-twentieth century social reform literature may note . . . a 'resolute refusal' to admit that individuals have any responsibility for their own stress."[12] Robert Whalen, Commissioner of the New York Department of Health, more explicitly makes the tie with high medical costs: "Unless we assume such individual and moral responsibility for our own health, we will soon learn what a cruel and expensive hoax we have worked upon ourselves through our belief that more money spent on health care is the way to better health."[13]

As do many advocates of individual responsibility, Walter McNerney, president of the Blue Cross Association, incorporates elements of both the Illichian and radical critiques of technology-heavy, distorted, and iatrogenic medicine: "We must stop throwing an array of technological processes and systems at lifestyle problems and stop equating more health services with better health . . . People must have the capability and the will to take greater responsibility for their own health."[14] John Knowles, the late president of the Rockefeller Foundation, spoke more directly to the problem of expectations: "The only thing we've heard about national health insurance from everybody is that it won't solve the problems. It will inflate expectations and demands and cause more frustrations."[15] Knowles argued that the "primary critical choice" facing the individual is "to change his personal bad habits or stop complaining. He can either remain the problem or become the solution to it: Beneficient Government cannot—indeed, should not—do it for him or to him."[16]

The attack on rights is explicit. Leon Kass, writing in *The Public Interest,* states that "it no more makes sense to claim a right to health than a right to health care."[17] "How can we go talking about a right to health," Robert Morrison asks, "without some balancing talk about an individual's responsibility to keep healthy."[18] Again, Knowles offers a clear articulation:

The idea of individual responsibility has been submerged in individual rights—rights or demands to be guaranteed by Big Brother and delivered by public and private institutions. The cost of sloth, gluttony, alcoholic intemperance, reckless driving, sexual frenzy and smoking have now become a national, not an individual, responsibility, and all justified as individual freedom. But one man's or woman's freedom in health is now another man's shackle in taxes and insurance premiums.[19]

What Knowles is suggesting by national responsibility is public policy aimed at changing individual behavior—and using economic or other sanctions to do it. Economic sanctions on individuals, such as higher taxation on the consumption of cigarettes and alcohol, or higher insurance premiums to those engaging in at-risk behaviors are becoming a popular theme. A guest editorial appeared last year in the *New York Times,* for example, introducing the idea of "Your Fault Insurance."[20] More extreme sanctions are proposed by Leon Kass:

> All the proposals for National Health Insurance embrace, without qualification, the no-fault principle. They therefore choose to ignore, or to treat as irrelevant, the importance of personal responsibility for the state of one's own health. As a result, they pass up an opportunity to build both positive and negative inducements into the insurance payment plan, by measures such as *refusing or reducing benefits for chronic respiratory disease care to persons who continue to smoke* [emphasis added].[21]

These sanctions may be justified under the rubric of "lack of motivation," "unsuitability for treatment," or "inability to profit from therapy."[22] Why waste money, after all, on people whose lifestyle contravenes good therapeutic results, or, as Morrison put it, on a "system which taxes the virtuous to send the improvident to the hospital."[23] In the new system the pariahs of the medical world and larger numbers of people in general could be diagnosed as lifestyle problems, referred to a health counselor, and sent home. At the very least, the victim-blaming ideology will help justify shifting the burden of costs back to users. A person who is responsible for his or her illness should be responsible for the bill as well.[24]

The Social Causation of Disease

If the victim-blaming ideology serves as a legitimization for the retrenchment from rights and entitlements, in relation to

255

the social causation of disease it functions as a colossal masque-rade. The complexities of social causation are only beginning to be explored. The ideology of individual responsibility, however, inhibits that understanding and substitutes instead an unrealistic behavioral model. It both ignores what is known about human behavior and minimizes the importance of evidence about the environmental assault on health. It instructs people to be indi-vidually responsible at a time when they are becoming less capable as individuals of controlling their total health environ-ment.[25] Although environmental factors are often recognized as "also relevant," the implication is that little can be done about an ineluctable, technological, and industrial society.

A certain portion of illness is, at some level, undoubtedly associated with individual behavior, and if that behavior were al-tered, it could lead to improved health. Health education efforts aimed at changing individual behavior should be an important part of any health strategy. Offered in a vacuum, however, such efforts will achieve only marginal results. Sociologist John Mc-Kinlay has argued convincingly that the frequent failure of health education programs is attributable to the failure to ad-dress the social context. He concludes that:

> Certain at-risk behaviors have become so inextricably intertwined with our dominant cultural system (perhaps even symbolic of it) that the routine display of such behavior almost signified member-ship in this society. . . . To request people to change or alter these behaviors is more or less to request the abandonment of dominant culture.[26]

What must be questioned is both the effectiveness and the political uses of a focus on lifestyles and on changing individual behavior without changing social structure and processes. Just as the Horatio Alger myth was based on the fact that just enough individuals achieve mobility to make the possibility be-lievable, so too significant health gains might be realized by some of those able to resist the incredible array of social forces aligned against healthy behavior. The vast majority, however, will remain unaffected.

The crisis of social causation is characterized by a growing awareness and politicization of environmental and occupational sources of disease in the face of the failure of medicine to have a significant impact on the modern epidemics, especially cancer.

In just the last few years the American people have been inundated with scientific and popular critiques of the environmental and occupational sources of cancer. These revelations have been accompanied by a constant flow of warnings about environmental dangers: air pollution, contamination of drinking supplies, food additive carcinogens, PCB, asbestos, kepone, vinyl chlorides, pesticides, nuclear power plants, saccharine, and even more. The Environmental Protection Agency, the Occupational Safety and Health Administration, and the Food and Drug Administration have been among the most embattled government agencies in recent years.

While there is considerable debate over threshold-limit values, the validity of animal research applications to humans, and specific policy decisions by the above agencies, awareness is growing that the public is being exposed to a multitude of environmental and work place carcinogens. Although many people still cling to the "it won't happen to me" response, the fear of cancer is becoming more widespread. A recent Gallup Poll found that cancer is by far the disease most feared by Americans, almost three times its nearest competitor.[27] The fear is not unwarranted. Cancer is a disease of epidemic proportions. Samuel Epstein, a noted cancer expert, claims that "more than 53 million people in the U.S. (over a quarter of the population) will develop some form of cancer in their lifetimes, and approximately 20 percent will die of it."[28]

Pressure on industrial corporations has been building for years. An occupational health and safety movement from within industry is gaining momentum. Many unions are developing programs and confronting corporate management on health and safety issues. Although suffering from severe setbacks, the environmental movement still poses a serious challenge as environmental consciousness is reinforced by the politicization of public health issues. Government agencies and the courts have never been so assertive, despite the repeated attempts by industry to undermine these efforts. The political constraints on the growth of the nuclear power industry and governmental pressures on steel are not lost on other industries.

The threat to corporate autonomy is clear. One reads almost daily of the economic blackmail threatened by corporations if regulations are imposed, whether production shutdowns, plant closings, or investment strikes. Corporations move their plants to more tractable communities or countries. Advertising campaigns promoting the image of public-spirited corporate activities attempt to counter the threat that the decision to subordinate people's health to profits will become yet more apparent. In short, the "manufacturers of illness" are on the defensive. They must seek new ways to blunt the efforts of the new health activists and to shift the burden of responsibility for health away from their doorstep.

The Politics of Diversion

Victim-blaming ideology offers a perfect opportunity. "For once we cannot blame the environment as much as we have to blame ourselves," says Ernst Wynder, president of the American Health Foundation. "The problem is now the inability of man to take care of himself."[29] Or as New York Health Commissioner Whalen writes: "Many of our most difficult contemporary health problems, such as cancer, heart disease and accidental injury, have a built-in behavioral component. . . . *If they are to be solved at all,* we must change our style of living" [emphasis added].[30] Alternatively, Leon Kass, fearing the consequences of a focus on social causation, warns of "excessive preoccupations, as when cancer phobia leads to government regulations that unreasonably restrict industrial activity."[31]

One after another, the lifestyle proponents admit to the environmental and occupational factors that affect health, but then go on to assert theri pragmatism. Victor Fuchs, for example, while recognizing environmental factors as "also relevant," asserts that "the greatest potential for reducing coronary disease, cancer, and other major killers still lies in altering personal behavior." He philosophizes that "emphasizing social responsibility can increase security, but it may be the security of the 'zoo'—purchased at the expense of freedom."[32] Carlson recognizes that social causation "raises some difficult political problems, because if we find the carcinogens in certain places in our environment, we run into institutional forces which will oppose dealing with them." Thus, "we may have to intervene at other levels here."[33] The practical focus of health efforts, in other words, should not be on the massive, expensive, politically difficult, or even politically dangerous task of overhauling our work and community environments. Instead, the focus must be on changing individuals who live and work within those settings. In the name of pragmatism, efficacy is thus ignored.

There are several other expressions of the ideology that should be noted. The diffusion of a psychological world view often reinforces the masking of social causation. Even though the psychiatric model substitutes social for natural explanations, problems still tend to be seen as amenable to change through personal transformation, with or without therapy. And, with or without therapy, individuals are ultimately held responsible for their own psychological well-being. Usually no one has to blame us for some psychological failure; we blame ourselves. Thus, psychological impairment can be just as effective as moral failing or genetic inferiority in blaming the victims and reinforcing dominant social relations.[34] People are alienated, unhappy, dropouts, criminals, angry, and activists, after all, because of maladjustment to one or another psychological norm.

The ideology of individual responsibility for health lends itself to this form of psychological obfuscation. Susceptibility to at-risk behaviors, if not a moral failing, is at least a psychological failing. New evidence relating psychological state to resistance or susceptibility to disease and accidents can and will be used to shift more responsibility to the individual. Industrial psychologists have long been employed with the intention that intervention at the individual level is the best way to reduce plant accidents in lieu of costly production changes. The implication is that people make themselves sick, not only mentally but physically. If job satisfaction is important to health, people should seek more rewarding employment. Cancer is a state of mind.

In another vein, many accounts of the current disease structure in the United States link disease with affluence. The affluent society and the lifestyles it has wrought, it is suggested, are the sources of the individual's degeneration and adoption of at-risk behaviors. Michael Halberstam, for example, writes that "most Americans die of excess rather than neglect or poverty."[35] Knowles's warnings about "sloth, gluttony, alcoholic intemperance, reckless driving, sexual frenzy and smoking," and later about "social failure," are reminiscent of a popularized conception of decaying Rome.[36] Thus, even though some

259

may complain about environmental hazards, people are really suffering from overindulgence of the good society; it is over-indulgence that must be checked. Further, by pointing to life-styles, which are usually presented as if they reflect the prob-lems of homogenized, affluent society, this aspect of the ideol-ogy tends to obscure the reality of class and the impact of social inequality on health. It is compatible with the conception that people are free agents. Social structure and constraints recede amid the abundance.

Of course, several diseases do stem from the lifestyles of the more affluent. Discretionary income usually allows for excessive consumption of unhealthy products; and, as Joseph Eyer argues, everyone suffers in variable and specific ways from the nature of work and the conditioning of lifestyles in advanced capitalist society.[37] But are the well-established relationships between low income and high infant mortality, diseases related to poor diet and malnutrition, stress, cancer, mental illness, traumas of various kinds, and other pathologies now to be ignored or rele-gated to a residual factor?[38] While long-term inequality in mor-bidity and mortality is declining, for almost every disease and for every indicator of morbidity, incidence increases as income falls.[39] In some specific cases the health gap appears to be widening.[40] Nonetheless, health economist Anne Somers re-assures that contemporary society is tending in the direction of homogeneity:

> If poverty seems so widespread, it is at least partly because our defi-nition of poverty is so much more generous than in the past—a generosity made possible only by the pervasive affluence and the im-pressive technological base upon which it rests. . . . This point—that the current crisis is the result of progress rather than retro-gression or decay—is vitally important not only as a historical fact but as a guide to problem solving in the health field as elsewhere.[41]

Finally, by focusing on the individual, the ideology performs the classical role of individualist ideologies in obscuring the class structure of work and the worker's lack of control over working conditions. The failure to maintain health in the work place is attributed to some personal flaw. The more than 2.5 million people disabled by occupational accidents and diseases each year and the 114,000 killed are not explained by the hazards

260

or pace of work as much as by the lack of sufficient caution by workers, laziness about wearing respirators or other protective equipment, psychological maladjustment, including an inability to minimize stress, and even by the worker's genetic susceptibility. Correspondingly, the overworked, overstressed worker is offered transcendental meditation, biofeedback, psychological counseling, or some other holistic approach to healthy behavior change, leaving intact the structure of employer incentives and sanctions that reward the retention of work place hazards and health-denying behavior.

Moreover, corporate managment appears to be integrating victim-blaming themes into personnel policies as health becomes an important rubric for traditional mangagerial strategies aimed at controlling the work force. Holding individual workers responsible for their susceptibility to illness or for their psychological state is not only a response to growing pressures over occupational hazards but it also complements management attempts to control absenteeism and enhance productivity. Job dissatisfaction and job-induced stress (in both their psychological and physical manifestations), principal sources of absenteeism and low productivity, will more and more become identified as lifestyle problems of the worker. Workers found to be "irresponsible" in maintaining their health or psychological stability, as manifest in attendance and productivity records, will face sanctions, dismissals or early retirement, rationalized as stemming from employee health problems. Already the attack on sick-day benefits is well underway. The push toward corporate health maintenance organizations will further reinforce managerial use of health criteria for control purposes.

One such control mechanism is pre-employment and periodic health screening, which is now in regular use in large industry. New businesses are selling employee risk evaluations, called by one firm "health hazard appraisals." Among the specific advantages cited for health screening by the Conference Board, a business research organization, is the selection "of those judged to present the least risk of unstable attendance, costly illness, poor productivity, or short tenure."[42] Screening also holds out the possibility of cost savings from reduced insurance rates and compensation claims. It also raises, however, the possibility of a large and growing category of "high-risk" workers who become permanently unemployable—not only because of existing, incapacitating illnesses but because of their *potential* for becoming ill.

In a period in which we have become accustomed to ozone watches in which "vulnerable" people are warned to reduce activity, workers are being screened for susceptibility to job hazards. Even though they alert individuals to their higher risks, these programs do not address the hazardous conditions that to some degree affect all workers. Thus, all workers may be penalized *to the extent* that such programs function to divert attention from causative conditions. To the degree that the causative agent remains, the more susceptible workers are also penalized in that they must shoulder the burden of the hazardous conditions either by looking for another, perhaps nonexistent, job; or, if it is permitted, by taking a risk in remaining. At a United Auto Workers conference on lead, the union's president summed up industry's tactics as "fix the worker, not the workplace." He further criticized the "exclusion of so-called 'sensitive' groups of workers, the use of dangerous chemical agents to artifically lower workers' blood lead levels, the transfer of workers in and out of high lead areas, and the forced use of personal respirators instead of engineering controls to clean the air in the workplace."[43] These struggles to place responsibility are bound to intensify.

A Policy Illustration

As previously noted, victim-blaming assumptions are already becoming a basis for the formulation of public policy. A good example is the area of health education. At a time when the health education profession needs to develop a new strategy that enlarges its focus "to include the political and social context in which the individual's health-related choices are being made," the individual-behavior orientation of the field has become more pronounced in response to the developments described in this article.[44] The recent Task Force on Health Promotion and Consumer Health Education, sponsored by the National Institutes of Health and American College of Preventive Medicine, for example, repeatedly emphasized a victim-blaming approach in its report. The Task Force made several policy recommendations overwhelmingly oriented toward the assumption of individual responsibility. The Task Force reasoned:

> In view of the overriding importance of individual behavior and lifestyles as major factors in the nation's unsatisfactory health status and ever-rising health care bill, CHE [Consumer Health Education] with its emphasis on education and motivation of the individual and better individual use of the delivery system, must now be recognized as a top priority in the national commitment to health promotion.[45]

Some members of the Task Force pressed for a different, more policy-oriented approach for health education. These concerns were acknowledged. The Task Force, nonetheless, made its priorities clear. In response to the appeal for the alternative orientation, the Task Force warned:

> However, there is also danger in pushing this view too far. Overemphasis on broad policy issues to the neglect of more traditional individual instruction could lead to loss of identity for health education as a profession. . . . If health education is to survive as a profession, rather than just a movement, or a philosophy of life, it must acquire more precise discipline.[46]

These remarks indicate that the Task Force members are keenly aware of the political constraints that impinge on the growth and prosperity of a profession. The remarks should also serve as a warning against placing too much faith in present health education efforts. While there are dissenting voices in the profession's hierarchy and probably many more among its rank and file, the profession seems bound to conceptions generated and sustained by political expedience. Indeed, a movement is precisely what is needed to free health promotion activities from professional and political control.

Similarly, the National Consumer Health Information and Health Promotion Act of 1976 is concerned almost exclusively with modifying individual health behavior and encouraging "appropriate use of health care." In providing support to community programs, for example, funding is mandated *only* for programs that promote "appropriate use" or "emphasize the prevention or moderation of illness or accidents that appear controllable through individual knowledge and behavior." In another section, the statute provides support for "individual and group self-help programs designed to assist the participant in using his individual capacities to deal with health problems. . . ."[47] The ideological themes noted in the Task Force report are now ensconced in law and constitute national policy.

Conclusion

On the one hand, America has become a society ridden with anxiety about disease and yet infatuated with the claims of scientific medicine. Access to medical services has come to be considered a basic right. These notions of rights have emerged from a long history of union and popular struggles negotiated in labor contracts and promoted through legislation. The campaign for national health insurance has gained a new vitality. In some quarters a national health service is being seriously considered; for example, the American Public Health Association endorsed the concept in 1977, and the bill was introduced in Congress by Representative Ron Dellums. On the other hand, the costs of medicine in the context of economic and fiscal crises are making services more difficult to obtain and are forcing a retreat from public programs. Corporate and governmental opposition to the extension of entitlements is becoming more pronounced.

At a time when people feel vulnerable to epidemic-proportion diseases, and powerless to do much about them, the tendency is to want medicine all the more. The great promise of the twentieth century will not be easily dispelled. Thus, when people want medicine the most, its continuing availability and expansion threaten powerful economic and political interests.

Further, in showing itself inadequate in dealing with contemporary disease, medicine is increasingly unable to perform its traditional function of resolving societal tensions that arise when people identify the social causes of their individual pathologies. The unique dilemma facing dominant interests is that people want both medicine and health, and the present social arrangements can give them neither. In the face of these trends, it is fascinating and revealing that we are witnessing the proliferation of a new ideology telling us that the problem is our individual lifestyles, that what we need is more individual responsibility for our own health.

Notes

1. For example, see B. Ehrenreich and J. Ehrenreich, "Medicine and Social Control," in *Welfare in America: Controlling the "Dangerous Classes,"* ed. by B. R. Mandell, (Englewood Cliffs, N.J.: Prentice-Hall, 1975), pp. 138-67.

2. T. McKeown, *Medicine in Modern Society* (London: G. Allen and Unwin, 1965); T. McKeown, "An Historical Appraisal of the Medical Task," in *Medical History and Medical Care: A Symposium of Perspectives,* ed. by T. McKeown and G. McLachlan (London: Oxford University Press, 1971), pp. 29-55; A. L. Cochran, *Effectiveness and Efficiency: Random Reflections on Health Services* (London: Nuffield Provincial Hospital Trust, 1972); J. Powles, "On the Limitations of Modern Medicine," *Science, Medicine and Man* 1, 1(1973): 1-30; I. Illich, *Medical Nemesis: The Expropriation of Health* (New York: Pantheon Books, 1975); V. Fuchs, *Who Shall Live? Health, Economics and Social Choice* (New York: Basic Books, 1974); R. Carlson, *The End of Medicine* (New York: John Wiley and Sons, 1975).

3. As described in one recent account, the holistic health movement believes that "disease is usually a stop sign, telling the individual to stop some process in life which is damaging to health. Disease is teacher." It includes therapies such as stress relaxation, polarity massage, meditation, nutrition, biofeedback, yoga, and dance. Upon joining one center, people are surveyed "on their relationship to their job and the significant persons in their immediate environment." They are "questioned on their time-management habits" and "asked if they perceive the world as hostile or friendly or indifferent" (*Chicago ·Sun-Times,* 11 December 1977, p. 104). See also *Conference on Future Directions in Health Care: The Dimensions of Medicine,* sponsored by Blue Cross Association, the Rockefeller Foundation, and the Health Policy Program, University of California, New York, December 1975.

4. Paul Starr, "The Politics of Therapeutic Nihilism," *Working Papers,* Summer 1976.

5. "The Use of Health Services by the Poor," *Social Policy* 5, 1(1974): 42.

6. *Chicago Sun-Times,* 16 March 1976.

7. "Inflation of Health Care Costs, 1976," hearings before the Sub-Committee on Health of the Committee on Labor and Public Welfare, United States Senate, 94th Congress (Washington, D.C.: U.S. Government Printing Office, 1976), pp. 656-60.

8. Daniel Fox and Robert Crawford, "Health Politics in the United States," in *Handbook of Medical Sociology,* edited by H. E. Freeman, S. Levine, and L. Reeder, (Englewood Cliffs, N.J.: Prentice-Hall 3rd. ed., 1979); Ronda Kotelchuck, "Government Cost Control Strategies," *Health-PAC Bulletin,* no. 75, March-April 1977, pp. 1-6.

9. *The Complex Puzzle of Rising Health Costs: Can the Private Sector Fit It Together?* (Washington, D.C.: Council on Wage and Price Stability, December 1976).

10. *New York Times,* 26 April 1977.

11.   The ideology of individual responsibility threatens to incorporate and use the self-help movement for its own purposes. Self-help initially developed as a political response to the oppressive character of professional and male domination in medicine. As such, the self-help movement embodies some of the best strands of grassroots, autonomous action, of people attempting at some level to regain control over their lives, and a response to the overmedicalization of American life. However, because the movement has focused on individual behavior and only rarely addressed the social and physical environment, and because it has not built a movement that goes beyond self-care to demanding the medical and environmental prerequisites for maintaining health, it lends itself to the purposes of victim-blaming. Just as the language of helping obscured the unequal power relationships of a growing therapeutic state (in other words, masking political behavior by calling it therapeutic), the language of self-help obscures the power relations underlying the social causation of disease and the dominant interests that now seek to reorder popular expectations of rights and entitlements for access to medical services.

12.   Fuchs, p. 27.

13.   *New York Times,* 17 April 1977.

14.   *Conference on Future Directions in Health Care,* pp. 4-5.

15.   Ibid., pp. 28-29.

16.   "The Responsibility of the Individual," in *Doing Better and Feeling Worse: Health in the United States,* ed. by John Knowles (New York: Norton and Co., 1977), p. 78.

17.   "Regarding the End of Medicine and the Pursuit of Health," *Public Interest* 40 (Summer 1975): 38-39.

18.   Quoted in ibid., p. 42.

19.   *Conference on Future Directions in Health Care,* pp. 2-3.

20.   14 October 1976.

21.   Kass, p. 71.

22.   William Ryan, *Blaming the Victim* (New York: Vintage Books, 1971).

23.   Quoted in Kass, p. 42.

24.   These remarks are in no way intended to imply that access to more services, regardless of their utility for improved health status, is a progressive position. Medical services as a means to maintain health have been grossly oversold. As Paul Starr comments, "a critic like Illich argues that because medical care has made no difference in health, we should not be particularly concerned about access. He has turned the point around. We will have to be especially concerned about inequalities if we are to make future investments in medical care effective" (p. 52). The argument here is that medical expenditures are presently distorted toward unnecessary and ineffective activities that serve to maximize income for providers and suppliers. Political conditions favoring an effective and just reallocation of expenditures are more likely to develop in the context of a publicly accountable system that must allocate services within statutory constraints and a politically determined budget. In such a system political struggles against special interests, misallocation, or underfunding will

obviously continue, as will efforts to achieve effectiveness and responsiveness. The concept and definition of need will move to the center of policy discussions. With all the perils and ideological manipulations that process will entail, it is better that such a debate take place in public than be determined by the private market.

Further, viable programs of cost control must be formulated, first as an alternative to the cutback strategy and, second, as the necessary adjunct to establishing effective and relevant services. Technology-intensive and over-use-related sources of inflationary costs are directly related to the problem of ineffectiveness as well as to iatrogenesis.

25. "Special Issue on the Economy, Medicine and Health," ed. by Joseph Eyer, *International Journal of Health Services* 7, 1(January 1977); "The Social Etiology of Disease, Part I," *HMO-Network for Marxist Studies in Health,* no. 2, January 1977.

26. "A Case for Refocusing Upstream—The Political Economy of Illness" (Boston University, unpublished paper, 1974).

27. *Chicago Sun-Times,* 6 February 1977.

28. "The Political and Economic Basis of Cancer," *Technology Review* 78, 8(1976): 1.

29. *Conference on Future Directions in Health Care,* p. 52.

30. *New York Times,* 17 April 1977.

31. Kass, p. 42.

32. Fuchs, pp. 26, 46.

33. *Conference on Future Directions in Health Care,* p. 116.

34. Thomas Szasz, *Ideology and Insanity: Essays on the Psychiatric Dehumanization of Man* (Garden City, N.J.: Doubleday-Anchor Press, 1970).

35. Quoted in Anne Somers, *Health Care in Transition: Directions for the Future* (Chicago: Hospital Research and Educational Trust, 1971), p. 32.

36. See note 19, above.

37. "Prosperity as a Cause of Disease," *International Journal of Health Services* 7, 1(January 1977) 125-50.

38. R. Hurley, "The Health Crisis of the Poor," in *The Social Organization of Health,* ed. by H. P. Dreitzel (New York :Macmillan, 1971), pp. 83-122; *Infant Mortality Rates: Socioeconomic Factors,* Washington, D.C.: U.S. Public Health Service, series 22, no. 14, 1972; *Selected Vital and Health Statistics in Poverty and Nonpoverty Areas of 19 Large Cities, U.S., 1969-71,* Washington, D.C. :U.S. Public Health Service, series 21, no. 26, 1975; E. Kitagaw and P. Hauser, *Differential Mortality in the U.S. : A Study of Socioeconomic Epidemiology* (Cambridge : Harvard University Press, 1973); Hila Sherer, "Hypertension," *HMO* no. 2, January 1977.

39. *Preventive Medicine USA* (New York: Prodist Press, 1976), pp. 620-21; A. Antonovsky, "Social Class, Life Expectancy, and Overall Mortality," *Milbank Memorial Fund Quarterly* 5, 45, no. 2-part 1 (1967): 31-73.

40. C. D. Jenkins, "Recent Evidence Supporting Psychologic and Social Risk Factors for Coronary Heart Diseases," *New England Journal of*

Medicine 294, 18 (1976): 987-94; and 294, 19 (1976): 1,003-38; J. Eyer and P. Sterling, "Stress Related Mortality and Social Organization," *Review of Radical Political Economy,* Summer 1977.

41. Somers, p. 77.

42. S. Lusterman, *Industry Roles in Health Care* (New York: National Industrial Conference Board, 1974), p. 31.

43. *Dollars and Sense,* April 1977, p. 15.

44. *Preventive Medicine,* pp. 171-72.

45. Ibid., p. 88.

46. Ibid., p. 24.

47. Public Law 94-317, Title I, 94th Congress, 23 June 1976.

Index

Abraham, Abraham, 112, 119, 124
Abrams, Herbert, 9
Ackerknecht, Erwin, 9, 11
American Association for the History of Medicine, 262
American College of Preventive Medicine, 262
American College of Surgery, 30
American Health Foundation, 258
American Hospital Association, 113, 208, 215
American Medical Association, 75, 79, 133, 139; Council on Medical Education, 133, 140, 141, 192; and demonstrative midwifery, 79-80; *Journal of the,* 127, 138, 188, 189, 191, 192, 193, 194, 195, 196; and reform of medical education, 140-41, 185-200 passim; Section on Obstetrics and Gynecology, 29
American Nurses Association, 212, 216, 219
American Public Health Association, 264
Anesthesia. *See* Twilight sleep
Anker, Frank, 9
Association of American Medical Colleges, 133
Asylums in ante-bellum Massachusetts, 156-78; determinants of death in, 173-76; English and French influences on, 157; epidemic death in, 165-67; super-

intendents' use of mortality statistics, 168-69, 172, 177-78
Axelrod, Sy, 9

Bacteriological practice, 120
Barker, Lewelly F., 137, 142
Bell, Luther B., 162, 163, 165, 167, 178
Bemis, Merrick, 177
Bevan, Arthur Dean, 140
Bigelow, Henry J., 109
Billings, F., 194
Blackwell, Elizabeth, 70
Blacks: medical education for, 143; in Montefiore work force, 231
Bloch, Jacques, 233, 235
Blue Cross Association, 249, 251, 254
Bluestone, E. M., 228
Bohack, H. C., 124
Boston City Hospital, 111, 114
Boston Dispensary, 109
Boston Medical Society, 110
Bowles, Thelma, 234
Boyd, Mary, 21, 22, 24, 28, 30
Breslow, Lester, 9
Brieger, Gert, 11
Brooklyn Hospital, 119, 120, 123, 124, 126, 128
Brooklyn hospitals, 118-28 passim
Brooklyn Maternity Hospital, 119
Burgess, May Ayres, 212
Butler, Nicholas Murray, 147, 148, 149

269

General Education Board. *See*
Rockefeller Foundation, General
Education Board
General Motors, 251, 152
Geneva Medical College, 70
Gilbreth, Frank, 209
Gilbreth, Lillian, 216, 218
Gleason, Ezra W., 56
Godoff, Elliot, 229, 232, 233, 236
Goldstein, Sarah, 240
Goodnow, Minnie, 216
Goodrich, Anne, 216
Green, Charles M., 20
Greene, Jerome D., 136
Grob, Gerald, 12
Gruenberg, Ernest, 9

Halberstam, Michael, 259
Hall, Diana Long, 133
Halsted, William S., 135, 142
Happel, T. J., 189
Harkness, Edward S., 148
Harrar, J. A., 23
Harvard Medical School, 143-45,
197
Health care system: access to, 8,
248, 253; growth of, 227, 228,
241, 248; political controversies
in, 8
Health education, 256, 262-64.
See also Ladies' Physiological
Institute of Boston and Vicinity;
Personal health
Health Insurance Plan of New York,
9
Health Policy Program of the
University of California, 249
Health reform movement of nine-
teenth century, 46-48, 74.
See also Ladies' Physiological
Institute of Boston and Vicinity;
Personal health
History of medicine, 3-12; and
medical education, 6-7; and
medical practitioners, 4-5, 6; and
the "new social history," 11-12
Hofstadter, Richard, 11
Hollick, Frederick, 56

Homeopathic Hospital (Brooklyn),
121
Hospitals: business rationalization
of, 123-28, 207-9, 218-19,
232-33; conversion from charity
to paying patients, 105-9, 117-
18, 120-23, 125-26, 208, 209;
financing of, 119-23; hierarchies
in, 230-31; internal organization
of facilities in, 126-27; maternity, 28-29, 31-32; nurses in
work force of, 207-8, 213-215;
private physicians and, 123-24;
rising costs at turn of century,
112-14, 118, 119-20; and urban
living patterns, 111; work force
in, characteristics of, 226-27,
230-31. *See also names of
individual hospitals*
Howell, Thomas, 112
Howland, Charles, 142, 144
Hunt, Harriet Kezia, 54, 56

Ideology: of individual responsibility, 250-51, 258-62; of
medical profession, 185; of
medical retrenchment, 254-
55
Illich, Ivan, 249
Immigration: and hospitals in late
nineteenth century, 107; to
Milwaukee, 85-86; and Montefiore Hospital work force, 230-
31
Insanity, 156, 157, 158-59, 163-66
Institute of the History of Medicine,
University of Leipzig, 7

Janeway, Theodore, 142
Janis, Lee, 9
Jefferson Medical College (Phila-
delphia), 71
Jewish Hospital (Brooklyn), 119,
124
Johns Hopkins Hospital, 33, 34
Johns Hopkins Hospital Historical
Club, 6
Johns Hopkins Institute of the